# The Spring Principle

## The Secrets to
## Dynamic Aging Revealed

# SUSAN SOFFER COHN

First published by Ultimate World Publishing 2024

ISBN

Paperback: 978-1-922714-98-5
Ebook: 978-1-922714-99-2

**Cover design:** Ultimate World Publishing
**Layout and typesetting:** Ultimate World Publishing
**Editor:** Rebecca Low

Ultimate World Publishing
Diamond Creek,
Victoria Australia 3089
www.writeabook.com.au

# Dedication

*This book is dedicated to Alicia who saved my life.*

# Contents

# Introduction

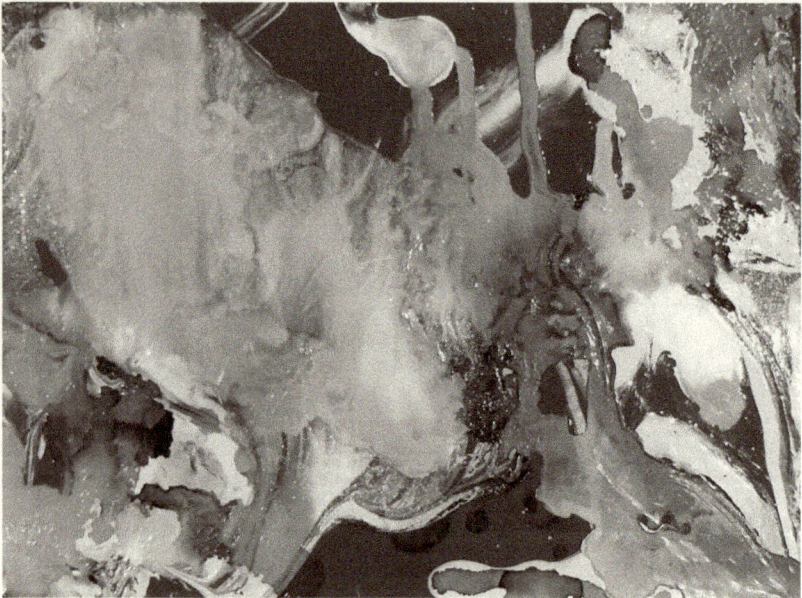

"Do one thing every day that scares you."

— Eleanor Roosevelt

S o, what's the significance of referring to spring when we're talking about aging? When we speak of the winters of our lives, we may think of the end of our days and a time of depleted energy and productivity. As the average life expectancy increases, we have been given a gift of time. We should consider how to use this time wisely rather than wasting it spending endless hours in front of a television, for example.

With these extra years, what are the possibilities? Are we going through the motions of living or challenging ourselves to live fully while we have days left on Earth? Thus, has what we used to call the winter of life become the new spring? As the population ages and we face many more years of living than we originally expected, we could be looking at a time of life that embodies creativity and adventures at the dawn of a new spring.

We have heard people say things like 50 is the new 30. For me, that isn't the most valid or important point regarding the principle of spring as it applies to looking at the later part of life in a new, positive way.

When we think about the season, spring tends to come earlier in the year. It is a season of growth, renewal, and regeneration.

As we look at an aging population that is looking at living longer and more dynamically, we can perhaps see spring in terms of regrowth and regeneration of our persona, our interests, our activities, our abilities in the area of creativity and insight, and our view of what a longer life may look and feel like.

We can take it to the next step of a springboard to growth. When we use a springboard, it gives us extra power and distance that we don't have when diving off the side of a pool. We can look at the extra years through the telescope of a new dawn of possibilities.

Think of a small stream of pure water flowing naturally from the earth. The extra years of life give us time to let the natural flow of creativity and wisdom flow through us to share with others.

Then, there's a device, such as a coil of wire. This device returns to its original shape after being compressed or stretched. Because of its ability to return to its original shape, springs are used to store energy, as in mechanical clocks, or lessen energy, as in the suspension system of vehicles. This can symbolize the storage of energy for productive purposes to provide the individual with a supply for growth in the time of the new spring of the Spring Principle.

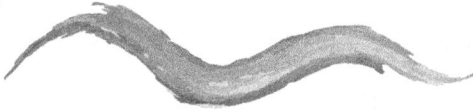

# SPRING

As we face challenges in the aging process, we will respond better if we have a model for figuring out our next step.

S... our model begins with gathering your **strength** to face the challenge of the day, week or moment. We are stronger than we know, and that awareness can give a sense of confidence.

P... we proceed to the next step of our model, **positivity**. A positive attitude can generally conquer any challenge. We need to believe we are strong enough and have the right attitude to get where we want to go.

R... carefully consider possible **responses** to the situation. List them and add pros and cons for each solution.

I... take **inspiration** from people and programs available nearby. Read, study, discuss and find out how others have handled a similar situation in the past.

N... list what you **need** in order to solve the problem.

G... solving a problem leads to **growth** in every situation. By facing life with gratitude and setting measurable goals, we continue to grow.

Remembering these steps keeps us on track for working through the constant issues we face as we age.

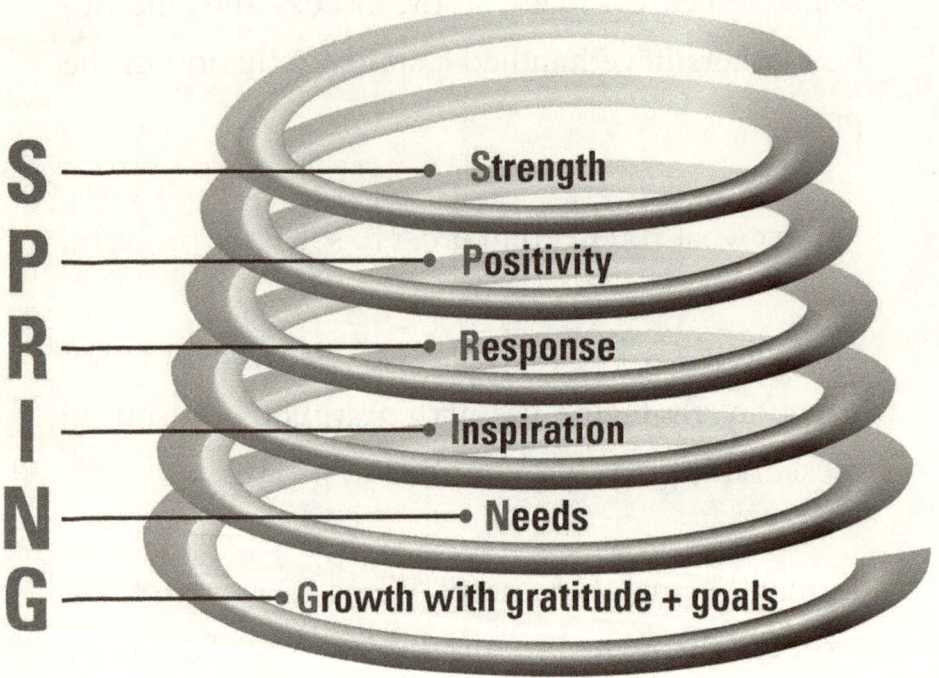

Strength

Positivity

Response

Inspiration

Needs

Growth with gratitude + goals

S
P
R
I
N
G

# So, What Does This Have to Do with Spring?

A spring is resilient, it is elastic, and it regains its original shape after removal from stress. Spring is a season of renewal; it's a source of clarity, the cool, clear running water from the earth. A springboard launches us into a wonderful action.

The more I looked at different definitions, the more I realized that these pieces of the word led themselves to the subject matter of this book in a way no other words could.

So, I am using these definitions to designate areas of the book and create a spring graphic with words for taking action as we set goals and make decisions for our futures.

If we use the spring formula as action steps for achieving our goals, it will help us focus on what is important to us as we proceed through life's stages.

We will use these steps:

S trength

P ositivity

R esponse

I nspiritation

N eeds

G rowth

Growth, Gratitude and Goals

# I Am Not Cute

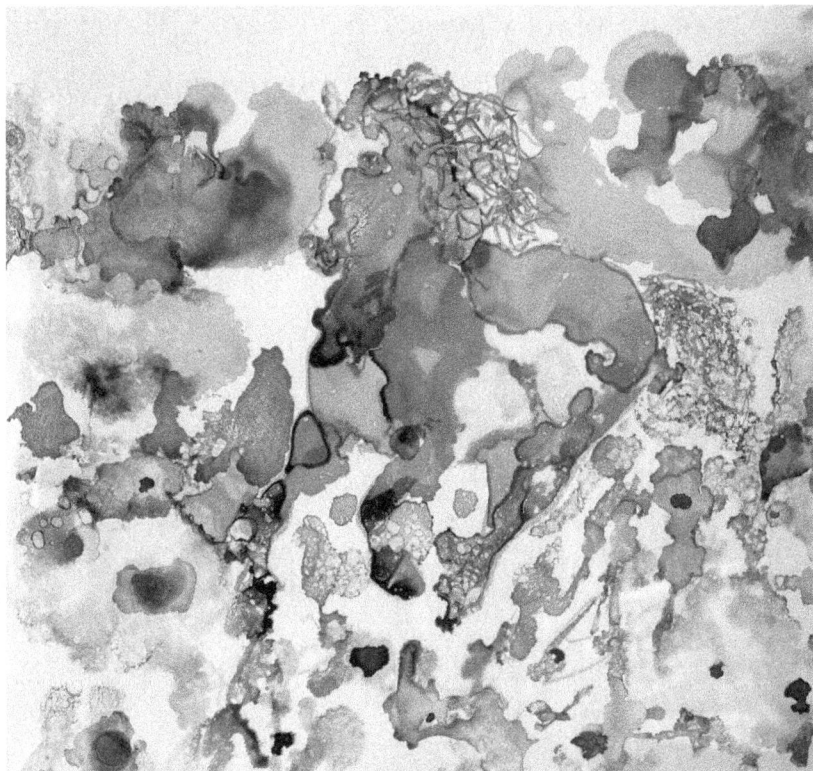

"Every year should be teaching us all something valuable. Whether you get the lesson is really up to you."
— Oprah Winfrey

# I Am Not Cute

What I am not:

I am not 80 years young. I have earned every day of my age, and it does not require exaggeration or hyperbole.

I am not cute. I have been called smart, attractive, and many other things, but never cute.

I am not a medical professional.

I am not an insurance agent.

I am not a Ph.D. candidate doing research.

I am an adult in my later years, who was married to another older adult for 57 years.

I am an adult human being with lots of life experience from all those years, but cuteness is not one of them.

I am not a poor old woman because I may be limping, or I may not be standing as straight as I once did.

I am not a little old lady because I lost inches and am not as tall as I once was.

I am Susan, proudly. My brain is working, as is my body. I am creative and challenge myself daily.

My work may be considered big, bold, experimental, dynamic, and/or innovative. It is not cute, sweet, or darling. I am an individual, inspired by proud artists, who does not aspire to cuteness, sweetness, or charm.

What I am: an educated 80-year-old woman, artist, author, and widow.

What I am not: stupid, demented, cute, a child, mute, deaf, or blind.

I read, I write, I paint, I love, I enjoy spending time with my friends, I live in my house, and I manage my affairs.

I paint daily without assistance from others. My work is not created by the observer but can enhance their environment.

If you use belittling phrases and apply them to my work, you belittle and insult the work, my being, my creativity, and all the hard work that goes into it.

I have friends and family going through the aging process with much discussion on an ongoing basis. I have watched parents and grandparents go through the process, and I have strong ideas, opinions, and impressions of how it is handled in the USA.

Though there are many people writing books about aging, I am hoping that my unique positioning will give another, perhaps unexplored aspect to be discussed, as well as inspiring dialogue among people of my generation and the ones to follow. This can enhance the ways we age in this country and the ways we deal with aging.

It is my hope to be part of the dialogue and to inspire others to get in on the thought process in order to share with those who come after us.

The huge difference today compared to 100 years ago is the average lifespan, which has as much as doubled.

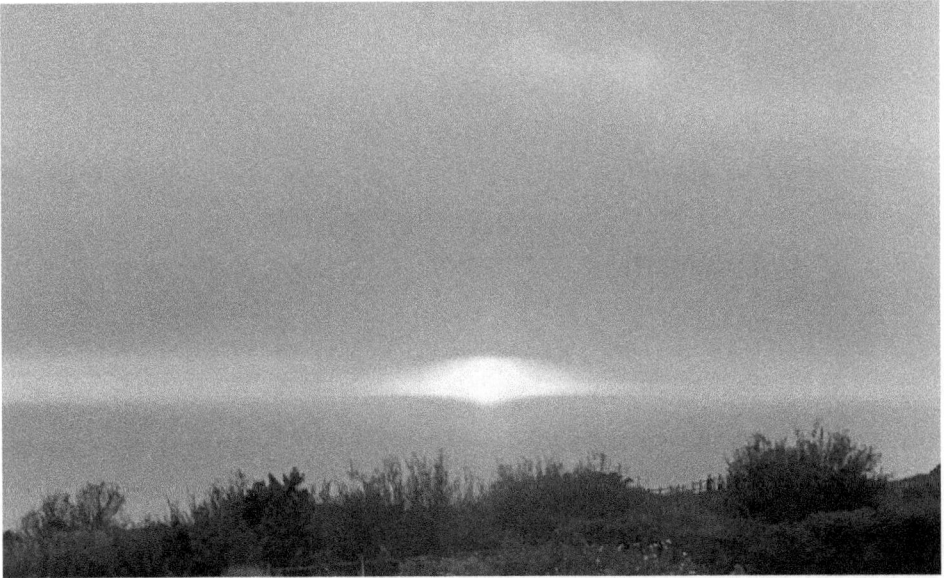

# My Panic Attack about Aging

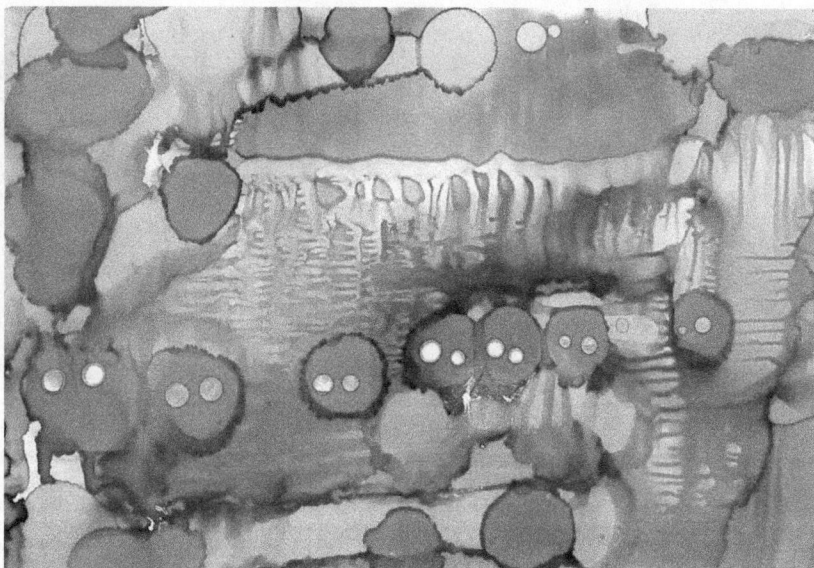

"Once I was beset with anxiety, but I pushed the fear away by studying the sky, determining when the moon would come out and where the sun would appear in the morning."
— **Louise Bourgeois**

It was my 50th birthday, and I had an appointment with my doctor for a physical. I walked to the office, and before I knew it, I was in tears. My children were grown; they had graduated from college and were on their way to having their own lives. My husband and I had spent the last 30 years of our lives working to earn the required income and have the time to provide them with life experiences to prepare them for adulthood.

Now, my husband Victor and I were trying to figure out what came next.

It seemed to me that day that it was all over. We had goals. We had reached them. The end. What now?

So, I met with my doctor in tears, trying to figure out what you're supposed to do when your life plan is over. He laughed at me (in a nice way). My doctor started telling me a story about a very young patient of his whose life was truly over, but faced each day with a positive attitude. What was he trying to tell me?

When I left his office that day, I was smiling, laughing at myself, and ready to face the world with whatever was coming next in my life. This was one doctor's visit that changed my life in a big way.

I stopped seeing my life as over.

I stopped seeing myself and my husband as old.

I stopped looking backwards and started looking forwards.

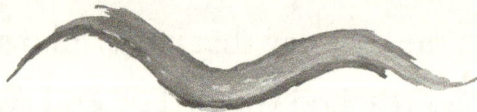

# Birthday Books... What Good Are They?

For my father's 85th birthday and my mother's 75th, my siblings and I planned parties to celebrate their lives, accomplishments, and relationships.

In each case, we sent out letters to friends and family telling everyone that we were celebrating and would like them to be part of it by submitting stories, photos, and other memorabilia. The responses were placed in albums, one for each of them, and they were truly remarkable.

What did I find the most interesting part? The lifelong relationships, stories, and the ability to share those stories with those fortunate enough to be able to attend the parties. Watching the joy on my parents' faces on these two occasions showed me how very important social connections are in a lifetime.

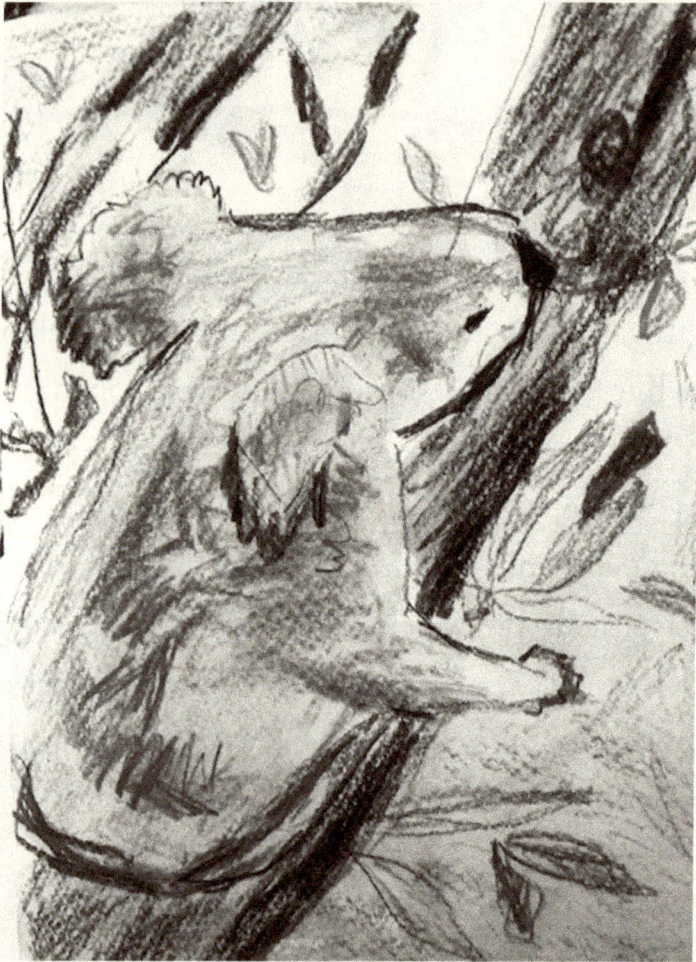

# The Infantilization of Elderly Persons: A Theory in Development

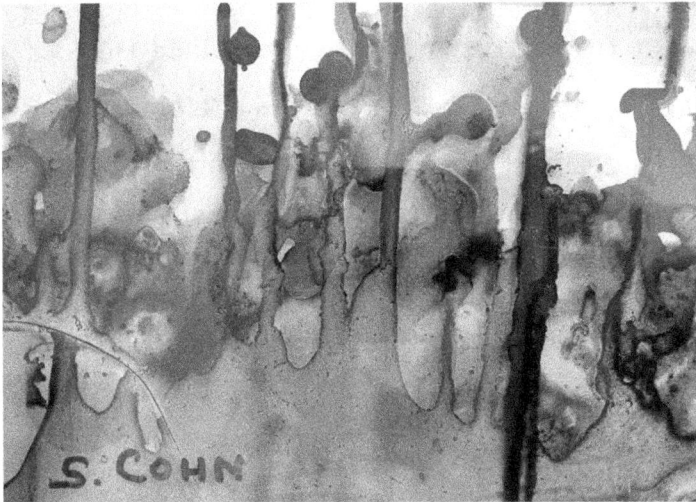

S. COHN

"I am old but I am forever young at heart. We are always the same age inside. Each year is special and precious. You can only live it once. Do not regret growing older. It is a privilege denied to many."

— Richard Gere

In a review of research on this subject, two North Carolina scientists pursued getting data for analysis from two companies run by people about the same age.

Two anecdotal situations piqued the researchers' interest. The first occurred in a nursing facility. The director of a nursing facility told of a well-liked, competent caregiver. She left the facility to pursue another opportunity and was replaced by a social worker who used a completely different approach with residents. The director of nursing (don) noticed a marked improvement in the verbal responses of the residents. The patients seemed more alert and less cognitively impaired in their interactions with staff and visitors.

The don noted that the only difference she could see was the differences in the caregivers' communication styles since both were caring staff members. In her attempt to be nurturing, the first caregiver spoke to the residents in a slow, sing-song voice using a childlike vocabulary. The caregiver who replaced her spoke to residents with the same adult speech patterns she used with staff.

Much to the surprise of the don, some residents who had previously spoken very little or who seemed to be showing signs of dementia started speaking and interacting in a normal way.

This anecdote caused the researchers to question whether infantilization alters the responses of elders to their caretakers and, in turn, increases the risk of the residents being labeled as cognitively incompetent.

A second incident occurred during a researcher's mother's last hospital stay as she was dying from cancer. She became quite angry with the nurses and doctors who infantilized her. She told them, "Just because I am old and can't hear you, don't think I'm stupid. Stop using baby talk with me and treating me like I'm not smart enough to make my own decisions."

This experience caused the researchers to ask whether elders considered infantilization a form of mistreatment.

Although college students and caregivers who hold stereotypes about the elderly consider baby-talk the most appropriate way to communicate with elders, most institutionalized elders view it as disrespectful and patronizing.

Language research shows that speakers tend to use accommodation strategies based on their assumptions of the listener's capability. Unfortunately, elders are often stereotyped.

Researchers Stephen M. Marson and Rasby M. Powell suggest that infantilizing and patronizing speech may be even more harmful to patients who don't protest. This acceptance, according to the study, creates a self-fulfilling prophecy by eliciting the expected behavior from the dependent elder.

## Questions:

Have you spoken to an older adult with baby talk?

_____

_____

_____

Have you been spoken to in slow speech or baby talk?

_____

_____

_____

What do you prefer to be called?

_____

_____

_____

What is an incident in your life when you have been made to feel stupid?

_____

_____

_____

_____

_____

_____

What could have been better?

_____

_____

_____

_____

_____

_____

# The Phone

————————

The phone rang a few minutes ago. It was the office of the home health agency that sends my physical therapist and a visiting nurse.

The woman on the other end of the phone said that the nurse told her I didn't answer the phone.

"I don't always answer the phone," I agreed. "I am working, and I am busy."

"What do you mean you are working!" she said in a confrontational manner.

"I am working," I repeated.

Just because I have had a couple of serious surgeries in the last few years that require follow-up and therapy does not put me out of the realm of being in the adult world, does it?

Who is making these assumptions? Who is trying to put me in my place (wherever they think that is)?

I was irritated that she jumped to whatever conclusion she had drawn about me. If I get health care, do I no longer qualify as a normal human being? What is it that she thinks I should be doing with my time when I am not answering the nurse's phone calls or working with a physical therapist twice a week? How am I to deal with this kind of assumption from a health care provider?

I was furious for lowering myself to offer an explanation for this woman, but I went on to posit what I might be doing when she decided I should answer the phone.

"I might be on another line or working on my latest book on my computer, or having a meeting with a prospective buyer, or organizing my work for yet another art show, or working intensely on a commissioned work of art for a client," I explained.

She was too startled that I would dare have anything more important to do than rush for the telephone whenever it rang, so I am certain what I said did not register with her in the slightest.

Have you had an experience similar to this one, during which someone made assumptions about what you could or should do with your time?

Expand on assumptions—what and where do they happen?

A list of assumptions:

- People assume that because of my age, I am not a successful artist and that I cannot produce work at this high level
- That I don't go to rock concerts
- That I am deaf
- That I can't see
- That I have dementia
- That, as an 80-year-old, I can't create something that would appeal to someone in their 20s or 30s
- That I don't want to have fun

# What is Ageism?

Ageism is stereotyping or discrimination against individuals or groups on the basis of age. The term was coined in 1969 by Robert Neil Butler to describe discrimination against seniors patterned on sexism and racism. Originally, this was geared chiefly towards older people, old age and the aging process. Ageism now includes biases that are part of institutional practices and policies which perpetuate stereotypes about elderly people.

## Employment

The concept of ageism was originally developed to refer to discrimination against older people. Mid-life workers, for example, often make more than younger workers do, which reflects achievement and experience. However, this often does not lead to a continued perception of high value as people advance beyond the middle years.

# Stereotyping

Stereotyping is a tool of cognition which involves categorizing people into groups and attributing characteristics to them. Stereotypes are good for processing large volumes of information that might be too large to give understanding to a group, even if the attributes can often be inaccurate.

When the content is incorrect with respect to a large number of people in a group, it can be harmful to develop these categories. For example, age-based stereotypes can prime an individual to draw significantly different conclusions when one sees an older or younger person with a similar limp. One might assume that the younger person's condition is temporary and treatable, while an older person's condition might be assumed to be chronic and less susceptible to intervention.

On average, this might be true, but plenty of older people have accidents and recover quickly, while young people could have an accident from which they become permanently disabled. This difference could be inconsequential when noting someone in a passing moment, but if it is held by a health professional offering treatment or managers thinking about occupational health, it could inappropriately influence their actions and lead to age-related discrimination and misdiagnosis.

Managers have been accused of stereotyping older workers as being resistant to change, not creative, cautious, slow to make judgements, lower in physical capacity, uninterested in technological change and difficult to train in similar management situations, which can lead to inappropriate management decisions.

A review of the research literature related to age discrimination in the workplace was recently published in the Journal of Management. Contrary to more obvious forms of stereotyping, such as racism and sexism, ageism is more resistant to change. For instance, if a child believes in an ageist idea against the elderly, fewer people correct them, and, as a result, individuals grow up believing in ageist ideas, even elders themselves. In other words, ageism can become a self-fulfilling prophecy.

Beliefs against the elderly are common in today's society. For example, an older person who forgets something could be quick to call it a "senior moment," failing to realize the ageism of that statement. People also often utter ageist phrases such as "dirty old man," or "second childhood," and elders can miss the ageist undertones.

Age discrimination exists in the USA. According to the EEOC, the first to complain were female flight attendants in 1968. That year, the EEOC declared that age restrictions for flight attendants were illegal discrimination under Title VII of the civil rights act of 1964. Yet Joanna Lahey at Texas A&M found that firms are 40% more likely to interview a young adult job applicant than an older one. Many sources place the blame on recruitment practices as it's the one way that age discrimination can go under the radar. People have a natural bias to hire someone like themselves. Since it is more difficult for workers to determine why they failed to receive an interview than why they have been fired, firms wishing to discriminate typically find it more beneficial to do so when hiring.

# Hollywood Ageism and Women

Profound ageism is seen in Hollywood, particularly in terms of women. This is seen from the way youth is praised and favored and the lack of opportunities for older women in film work. In a presentation on the subject, O. Burtch Drake stated, "Older women are not being portrayed at all; there is no imagery to worry about."

Women over 50 are not the center of attention, and if an actress is older, they are expected to act anything but their age. The standards set for women in film focus on youth, sexuality, and beauty. Films that feature older women acting their age seem exaggerated and unrealistic in the Hollywood environment because this does not fit the established norms associated with women in film and other media. As a result, women often find weak employment opportunities.

Due to the limited age the film industry shows and the lack of older actresses, society has a certain illiteracy about sexuality and those of old age. There becomes an inherent bias regarding what women are capable of, what they do and how they feel. In the case of actresses of all ages, there becomes an effort to maintain youthful looks and high beauty standards by altering themselves, including many plastic surgeries. In this way, frightened women in the industry worry about showing any signs of aging. In terms of sexuality, older women are shown as unattractive, bitter, unhappy, and unsuccessful in films. This can cause depression, anxiety and self-esteem issues. So, when a woman is told she is old, she can start to believe she is. She may start acting as if she is older due to internalizing what others say.

# Ageism in Healthcare

There is a large body of evidence of discrimination against the elderly in healthcare. This is particularly true in the patient/physician relationship. Studies have found that physicians seem to show significantly less care in trying to cure older people than younger ones. For example, health professionals tend to pursue less aggressive treatments for older patients. It has been suggested that this is because doctors fear their older patients are not strong enough to tolerate curative treatments; therefore, there is no point in trying to reverse the inevitable. Thus, approaches to treating older people tend to be concentrated on managing diseases instead of providing a cure or treatment.

Other research studies have shown there is an assumption that age inhibits healing; therefore, it's a waste of energy to try to reverse the inevitable. In addition, caregivers undermine the treatment of our elderly by helping them too much and treating them as feeble, which decreases their independence.

# Elderspeak

My grandmother, Gretchen Hess Braufman, was born in the state of New York near the end of the 19th century. She had one older brother who died quite young, at which time she became the oldest of what became eight siblings, all born in the USA. She was not "cute" or naïve or helpless. These words, which are often used to describe babies, had nothing to do with my grandmother. She was president of a local chapter of an international philanthropic organization for many years and ran a profitable business. She was widowed at a young age and had two young daughters.

She lived by herself in a nice apartment and had a housekeeper helping her who kept the house and did the cooking while my grandmother was at work. She died at age 92, only a year or two after she stopped driving. She was not in an institution, and she was not subject to employees who might treat her in a childlike way. As the matriarch of our family, no one would have considered talking down to her. My grandmother's house was the family lending library. When we went there for dinner, everyone brought their latest completed book and traded it with other members of the family.

In today's world, the term elderspeak has come into usage. It refers to the way that some people treat the elderly. It involves speaking more slowly and/or loudly, overenunciating words, and simplifying speech patterns. In addition, when asking an older person a question, the 'you' pronoun is replaced with a 'we,' implying that the older person cannot think or respond for themselves.

For example: "Are we enjoying our food today? I see that we are drinking tea, which we love, right?"

By asking the question without looking for a verbal response, the questioner makes an assumption that the senior is confused and does not have full cognition. However, health experts have noticed that this demeaning type of language may have a derogatory impact.

Dr. Becca Levy, a psychology and epidemiology professor at Yale University, has done some significant research on this topic. Dr. Levy told a New York Times reporter in an interview that her research indicates: "Those who have more negative images of aging in their lives have worse functional health over time, including lower rates of survival."

Professor Levy conducted a long-term study with 660 people over the age of 50. She discovered that when subjected to elderspeak and negative perceptions of their future, the participants lived an average of seven and a half years less than those with a positive feeling about aging who were not confronted with elderspeak. Her findings remained even after removing various factors to control health conditions.

One of the problems is that many people do not recognize that they use elderspeak, and if they did, they would likely not see anything wrong with it. However, the elderly experience this behavior as condescending, and they are exposed to it, not only in nursing facilities but in grocery stores, doctor's offices and restaurants. Though many do not openly oppose being "sweetied" and "honey'd", many take it as a personal insult.

In an article about Becca Levy's research, writer Kara Nihm stated that when she neared 70-plus years, she would: "Not want to be disregarded as a person who cannot think or do for herself. So before we thoughtlessly speak to senior citizens as if they are helpless, it's best to remember what our parents have always preached—always respect your elders."

What can we do about it?

The answer is: age should have no bearing on human dignity and respect. Seniors want to be recognized for who they are, not their age.

We read about ancient societies in which an old wise person is looked to for wisdom, insight, and depth. Unfortunately, in too many cases, our society has shifted to treating our older population as an inconvenience. It has become common practice to treat them as though they are young children. But why would we speak baby talk to young children and not show them the respect of teaching them our language as it should be spoken. This is a plea for treating all people with equal respect no matter their age.

We are infantilizing our seniors by treating them with condescension, as if they are mascots rather than people. You may not realize you have done it, but every time you see an elderly couple holding hands and say, "They're soooo cute," that's treating them as a mascot.

So, to summarize:

- Dignity at any age is the cornerstone of human existence.
- Our treatment of elders can impact their health.
- Disrespectful speech makes them feel incompetent.

- It can cause cognitive problems.
- Elderspeak is a form of bullying.
- Older adults want to be recognized for who they are, not their age.
- Talk to older adults about normal things. For example, over 80% of 50 to 90-year-olds are sexually active, yet we don't talk about it.

Becca Levy is credited with creating the field of how age stereotypes, which are assimilated from the culture, impact the health of older adults. The dean of the Columbia School of Public Health describes Levy as a "pioneer" in the growing body of impressive research showing that our attitudes toward aging affect our health, our resilience in the face of adversity, and our very survival.

Levy has created an area of research that focuses on the extent to which the aging process is a product of society. She has examined this in a series of innovative studies that demonstrate that culture-based positive and negative age stereotypes of older persons have beneficial and detrimental influences on a wide range of health conditions.

Studies have found that age stereotypes contribute to physical outcomes such as longevity, cardiovascular events, stress levels, and the will to live.

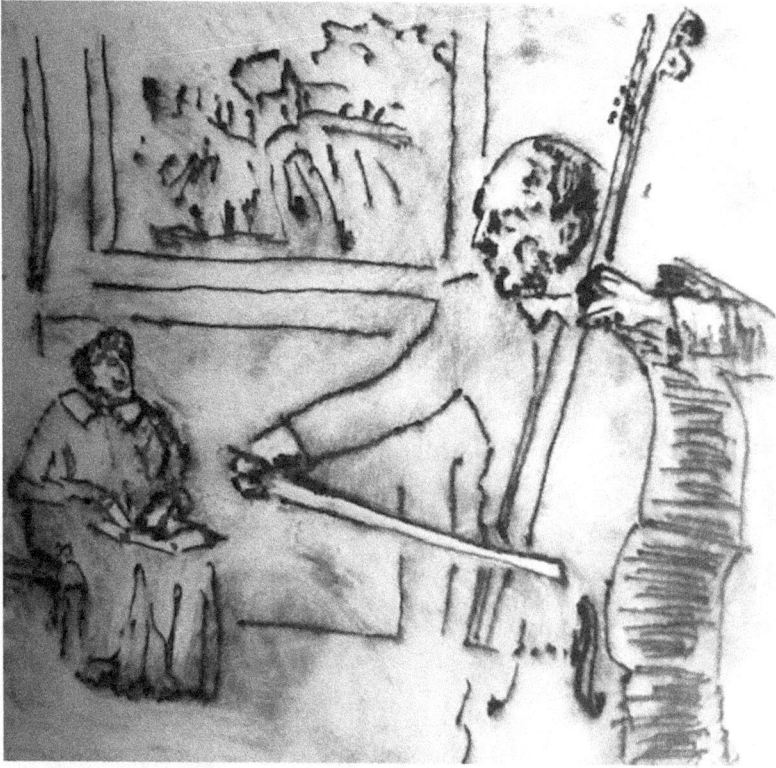

# 100 Years

"You've got to be a fool to want to stop the march of time."
— Pierre-Auguste Renoir

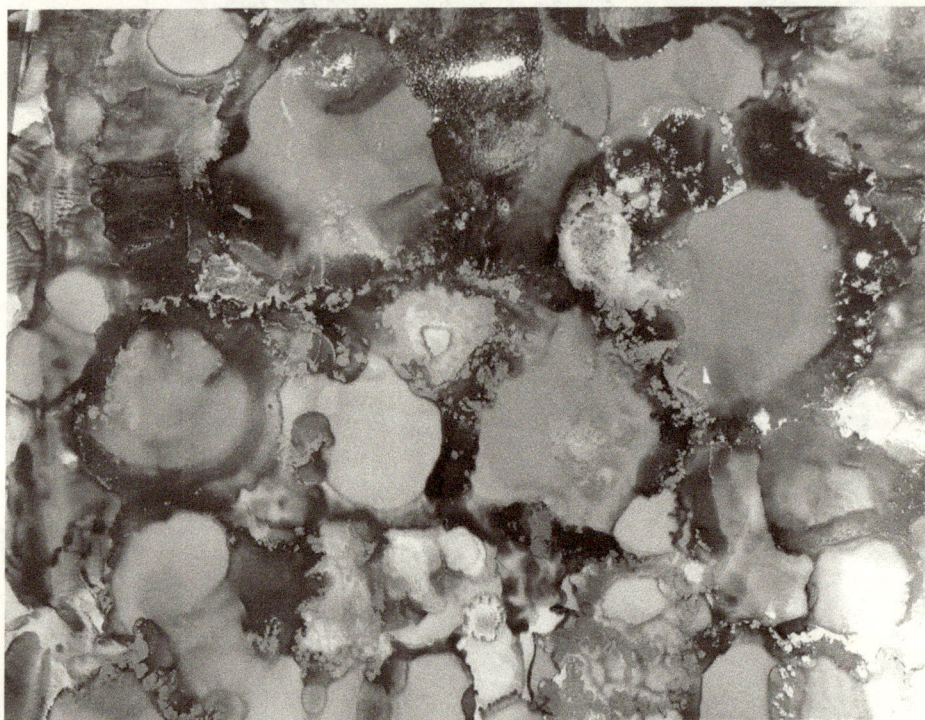

# 100 Years Old

Have you ever been to a 100-year-old's birthday party? I have been to three in recent years.

My favorite party was celebrating centenarian Sy Breen. The party had been planned at a restaurant on Palm Canyon Drive in Palm Springs on the second floor. They did not have an elevator.

Sy came bounding up the stairs at full speed and proceeded to visit each table full of friends and family, greeting everyone by name and chatting with each party goer.

An extraordinary man, Sy had been in television commercials, trained racehorses because of his small size, and owned a camera store. On his 90th birthday, he decided he was going to raise money to make mammograms available at no charge to women in the Coachella Valley.

He asked friends and family to sponsor him in a golf challenge. He planned to play 90 holes of golf on his 90th birthday and get people to pledge any amount per hole to go to his fund. On his birthday, friends came to the golf course to cheer him on, and Sy collected the pledges for the entire 90 holes he played that day. He went on for the next nine birthdays, adding eight more holes until he reached 99 holes in one day on his 99th birthday.

Sy, at 81, was the oldest person in the state of California to be approved as an adoptive parent. He had a young grandchild whose mother was not able to take care of him. He applied to adopt the child and was determined to raise him as his own until he was legally an adult. He did exactly that.

He was a hands-on parent, creating yearbooks for the child's classes on his computer. He also drove the boy to and from school every day.

He had a younger wife, who he loved to take dancing. We often accompanied them for dinner and dancing. They were nimbler and danced with more enthusiasm than my husband and I did, though we were decades younger.

The second 100th birthday party I attended honored my mother-in-law, Anne Cohn, who lived until just before her 107th birthday.

Anne Rudin Cohn was a very beautiful woman, an only child of Bessie Belsky and Jacob Rudin.

She grew up spoiled by both parents in a not-very-great marriage. She was the center of their lives and the apple of their eyes.

In her late teens, she met an attractive young man on the streets of South Haven, Michigan, and a few days later, they eloped. When she told her parents, they insisted that she come home immediately and have a proper courtship and marriage. That is why my in-laws had two wedding anniversaries each year: the day they thought they got married and the day their parents had a wedding for them and considered them officially married.

Leonard Cohn died at 89, but hardy Anne lived on. She exercised every day and ate a simple, healthy diet of natural foods. When she was 90 years old, she had hip replacement surgery. Three weeks later, she was driving again.

She always wanted a daughter and complained that she only had three sons. Anne loved having granddaughters and stayed as close to them as they would allow.

She ran a business from her desk in her home, keeping her mind active until she started to get lonely and bored late in her 90s. So, she moved to a facility that had social activities and started running the bingo game.

She was doing so well at 99 that the family decided to hold a birthday party as she was almost 100. That was the beginning of a series of years celebrating birthdays since who knew if there would be another coming.

There is a family photograph indicating the celebration of 105 years. If you count the fingers in the photo, they will add up to 105.

At these birthday parties, she loved to stand up as the center of attention and give long speeches to and about everyone in the family.

The third 100th birthday party I attended was for the father of a friend, Harry Kahan, who lived to be 103.

In his 90s, Harry Kahan went to the office in the morning. He was a CPA. He then drove to the Sand and Sea Club for lunch and sunshine. When the Sand and Sea Club closed for good, Harry was invited to join the Jonathan Club for his afternoon sunshine.

Harry's daughter, Nancy, invited us to join them for Harry's 100th birthday party. It was a beautiful day. He was no longer driving but was dressed well with a big smile on his face for the celebration.

With a little assistance, he stood at the appropriate time and made a beautiful speech, welcoming friends and family to the special occasion of his 100th birthday.

So, if I have been to three 100th birthday parties, there have to statistically be many more centenarians in this country and around the world.

There has been a huge increase in life expectancy in the last 100 years. One of my favorite books is, *I've Decided to Live 120 Years* by Ilchi Lee, which proposes that living to 120 is not very far off, considering the life span of many people already surviving well beyond 100 who are still productive and active.

His premise is that making the decision to live longer makes your life more productive while you are alive, no matter what age you live until.

There are currently so many 100th birthday parties that I found a website devoted to planning them with special products for the occasion.

# Attitudes on Aging

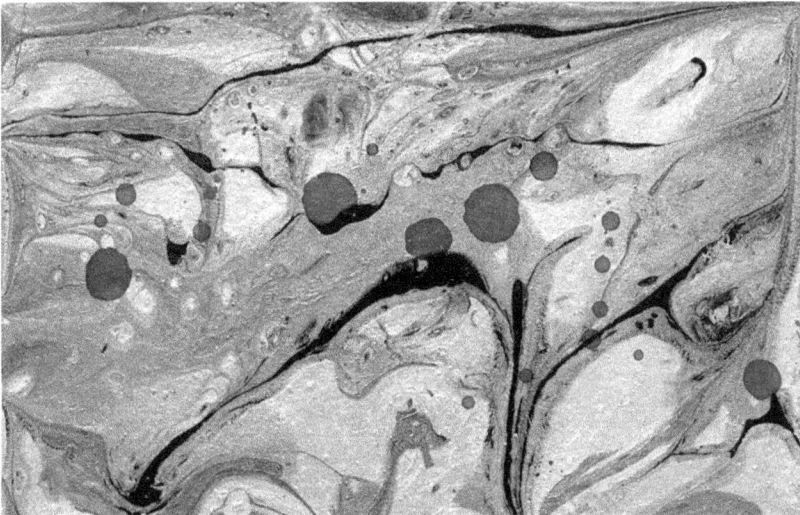

"We don't stop playing because we grow old. We grow old because we stop playing."
— George Bernard Shaw

Looking for comments on the internet is often a good way to find honest opinions and input on a subject. The following six sections include individuals talking about their attitudes on aging. I have included them to enhance the commentary of the included chapters.

## Fred the Veteran

**I'm 80.**

So, I'm old by almost every standard.

Mentally, I feel like I leveled out at 35. I have not been able to improve my chess score since then.

My stamina is down compared to 35, but no worse than it was when I was 50.

I still have all of my hair and teeth, and I can still wear the uniform the Air National Guard issued me in 1990. I have worn glasses since I was six, but my prescription has not changed since 2010. I have tinnitus resulting from going under an F-4 aircraft while both engines were running to remove or replace the 'remove before flight' flags. But it hasn't gotten worse since I was diagnosed in 1993.

Over the years, I have managed to dislocate both shoulders, so they don't work as well as they should. I have an umbilical and right inguinal hernia that causes me no discomfort.

In 2000, I was told I had prostate cancer and had to have an immediate operation. I declined, and it turned out to be a false positive. I have had a BPH since I was 35. I'm taking Tamsulosin for that, but when I forget to take it, it doesn't seem to make much difference. My wife reminds me if it slips my mind.

My libido hasn't decreased since I was 35. (My wife keeps asking, "When are you going to start acting your age?")

I DO eat bacon, butter, eggs, milk, real cream, cheese, raw nuts, salt, and fatty meat. I eat foods fried in coconut oil and eat olive oil in salad dressing as the only other oil. I drink a LOT of coffee. I eat raw and steamed fruits and vegetables, a high protein vegetable-based diet, with four ounces of meat per meal (optional).

I take a multivitamin, fish oil minerals, and Vitamin D3. My BP is 135 over 85, up from 120 over 80 five years ago. My cholesterol is 210 (unchanged since I was first tested at 18), LDL is low, triglycerides are low, mostly HDL.

I sleep like a rock, usually from 10 pm until 6 am, with a pee break around 4 am. If my sleep is interrupted, I take a short nap around 3 pm. I'm almost never sick, which is a good thing since my doctor dropped me (he had too many Medicare patients under the ACA). We have Medicare and Tricare-for-life, which should pay for almost everything. I do low-impact exercise daily and try to limit my sitting to under four hours per day. So much interesting stuff to learn, so little time.

I have been married to the same woman for 50 years now, and we're very compatible. I work to keep her happy. Her family thinks I've brainwashed her.

We raised two boys. They're in their 40s now.

I don't do drama. The last time anyone tried (my daughter-in-law), I rejected her drama with verbal military emphasis. She called me a horrible, fouled-mouth monster. I think she learned new words and hasn't been back. I didn't use any of George Carlin's seven banned words, either. She was already proficient with those. She went home to live with her mama, another drama queen. She attempted character assassination, telling everybody I was a mean SOB who hurt little kids when nobody was looking. I don't think anybody believed her, and if they did, too bad for them. **I believe the things that age you are infections, bad diet, lack of exercise, and emotional stress.**

I have always had fun jobs. Most recently, I've been a self-employed biomedical equipment repair person. I'm still working part-time in the biomedical field. However, everything I know about biomedical science will be obsolete within five years.

You can do a lot of stuff in 60 years. In South Florida, I was unemployed for two years (thank you, Jimmy Carter). We had no car, lived in a 10-year-old paid-for mobile home, and I picked up cans to buy grocery money. We ate a lot of fish during those two years.

I'm back into amateur radio and emergency communications, and volunteer for the Community Emergency Response Team. I've completed a boatload of Homeland Security correspondence courses. I keep chickens and a small garden. I'm working on learning permaculture and aquaponics.

**STAY ACTIVE. IF YOU DON'T USE IT, YOU LOSE IT (SERIOUSLY)!**

# Yayoi Kusama

Born in March 1929, Kusama started drawing pictures of pumpkins in elementary school. Her mother was supportive of her creative endeavors.

Her mother often sent her to spy on her father, who was having extramarital affairs, which turned her off when it came to interest in sex, it is said.

When Kusama was 10 years old, she began to have hallucinations. These included flowers, flashes of light, and dense fields of dots. These patterns have been carried forward in her art to this day.

Currently, in her 90s, Kusama is a force in the international art community. Her large installations can be seen in museums throughout the world. In 2017, a 50-year retrospective of her work opened at the Hirshhorn Museum in Washington, D.C. The exhibit featured six of her infinity mirror rooms which were scheduled to travel to five museums in the US and Canada.

The exhibit was temporarily closed due to a sculptural element in one of the rooms being destroyed. According to a museum official, the Hirshhorn has never had such high attendance for another exhibit as it did for Yayoi Kusama.

# Setting Lobster Traps at 101

Max Oliver is still working on a lobster boat at the age of 78, but that is not the astounding story. His crewmate and mother, Virginia, is 101 years old, still working on the ship three days a week from May to November, catching lobsters off the coast of Maine.

Together, the mother and son face the hazardous challenges of trapping lobsters, which she has been doing since childhood.

"It's not hard for me," she told the Boston Globe. "It might be hard for someone else, but not for me."

When asked how long Virginia plans to be lobstering, she indicates she has no interest in retiring. When someone asks how long she plans to work, she says, "Until I die. And I don't know when that will be."

# Ruth Salton at 100

It was the eve of her 100th birthday in January 2022, and Ruth Salton insisted on going to Friday night services at her Congregation Beth Israel. It was only days after a gunman spouting antisemitic lies held four hostages, worshipers, for 10 hours at the synagogue near Fort Worth, Texas.

As a Holocaust survivor, Salton insisted that she wanted to "support her people" by going to the synagogue. She determined that if her daughter didn't want to take her, she would get there somehow.

She said, "I'll go by myself because I belong there. I am Jewish, and this is my faith, and I am supporting it."

Salton was not the only one who felt the need to stand for what she believed in. A New York rabbi, Angela Buchdahl, stated, "A terrorist tried to steal Shabbat (the Sabbath) from us last week. Claiming it this week is an act of resistance."

In fact, at synagogues throughout the USA, members of congregations marked the week after the hostage-taking by attending en mass, with a show of defiance against the standoff and other acts of antisemitism. Many called for a large turnout to show unity among the faithful.

Having survived the Holocaust and more, Salton said she was ready to survive her centennial. Though she joked she might rather be 18, she said she was grateful to be celebrating her 100th birthday in a meaningful way, protesting hate.

# Los Angeles Times, November 28, 2021

Swimming into her second century, Maurine "MO" Kornfeld has qualified to swim competitively in the 100 - 104 age bracket as of January 1, 2021. She has received six world records since then, and she didn't begin competitive swimming until she was 60 years old.

Kornfeld is one of the oldest master swimmers in America and has outlived much of the competition to achieve her recent records. She reacts to her achievements with a certain degree of modesty. According to her coach, there is no boasting; it's all a matter of fact. Mo will say, "I got my best time, and I got a record. That's nice."

"I can't say it is anything particular about me," Kornfeld told an LA Times reporter in an interview. "Except that I have been very fortunate."

She gestures around her cozy Hollywood bungalow as she comments, "Look around you. I have everything I need."

## Faith Ringgold: Story Quilts

Another memorable artist was Faith Ringgold who sadly passed away this year aged 93. Ringgold was the recipient of the Smithsonian Craft Show's 2017 Visionary Award.

Ringgold is best known for painted narrative quilts inspired by Buddhist tankas—painted and brocaded fabric pictures. In the early 1970s, she abandoned traditional oils for paintings on acrylic on unstretched canvas and fabric borders.

She has been painting her signature story quilts ever since. Her work focuses on civil rights, gender equality, African American life and culture, family joys and hardships, and the education of children.

# Great Aunt Ruth

My great-aunt Ruth Hess worked in my grandmother's store as the buyer for her store and other stores of her siblings. When my grandmother retired and sold her store to a cousin, Aunt Ruth went to work for Uncle Henry in his clothing manufacturing business.

One day, she was walking across the busy street to my grandmother's, and a speeding car ran into her. She was taken to the hospital. We were told she would never walk or work again.

One fantastic woman, she was determined to do both, and within a few weeks, she was walking and working as a designer's consultant in the factory. After a few weeks, she didn't even limp and continued to wear the high heel wedge shoes she loved throughout her life.

# My Cousin Hans

My cousin, Hans Feist, escaped from Germany during WWII, as did his sister and brother. His brother Herbert made it to the United States, where he attended high school with my mother.

Hans renamed himself Chanan when he and his older sister arrived in Israel.

All three of the siblings got married, had children, and built lives in their new home countries.

Chanan was an extraordinary man. He earned a Ph.D. when he was in his 90s. His research project was an extensive family tree, including many branches of our family. As he researched the material, he was in touch with many family members all over the world.

The last time I got to spend time with him was on a trip to Israel. I had a party for family members and sat next to cousin Chanan. That evening, he told me family secrets I had never heard before.

One story emphasized the emigration of my great-grandparents. My great-grandfather had traveled from Lithuania to Germany to study. He met my great-grandmother, who was studying as well. She brought him home, and Chanan claims their parents were not happy with the match, but they were married just the same.

My great-grandfather had to check in with the government regularly. One year, he was told he had to leave the country. By this time, he had a wife and a baby boy. In shock, he got a ticket to America and promised my great-grandmother he would send for her and the boy, but he didn't. At last, her brothers traveled to America to search for their brother-in-law. In time, they found him, then they sent for their sister and reunited the couple in the new land.

# My Aunt Geri

My Aunt Geri lived next door to us. She loved introducing me to great music and literature. She would rush in the door and exclaim, "You need to come hear the new Rachmaninoff record I just bought."

As I listened, she would make comments like, "Isn't it powerful?"

She also enjoyed taking me to her annual group meeting, where each year, she presented a paper, introducing me to intellectual pursuits.

As I write this, she died two days before her 100th birthday but during her 99 years, she was as sharp as ever. I loved to visit her for good conversation.

# What Does It Feel Like to be Old?

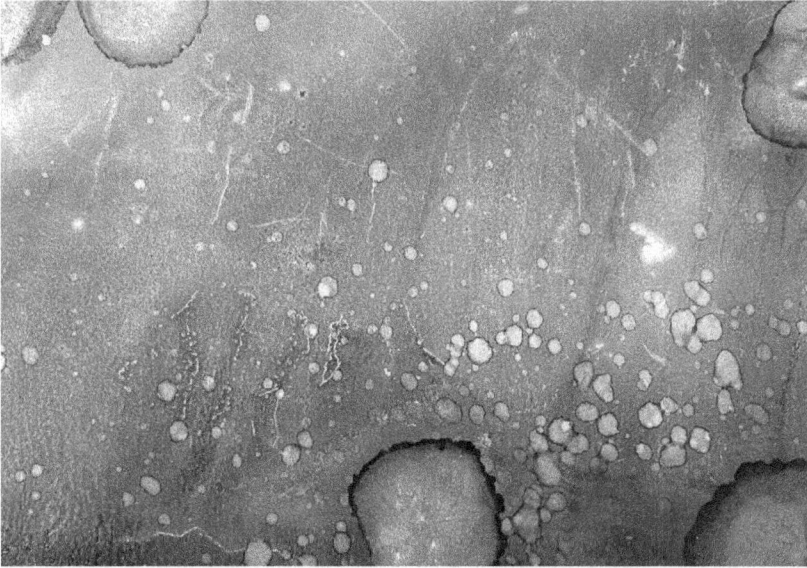

"I have found that every time I've made a radical change, it's helped me feel buoyant as an artist."
— David Bowie

# What Does It Feel Like to be Old?

## Add your own story and perspective.

_____

_____

_____

_____

_____

_____

_____

_____

_____

_____

_____

_____

_____

_____

# Do Old People Miss Being Young?

Oh my goodness, yes, we miss being young! When I was young, I never thought about being old. I guess I thought I would be young forever. It was as though one day, I woke up and couldn't do the things I used to do. My body ached, and everything hurt. I couldn't hear.

Everything became such an effort. I even stopped sitting on the floor with my dog or playing games with my grandkids because it was too hard to get up. I used to love to take baths, but I stopped because it's too hard to get out of the tub. People call me honey, sugar, and sweetheart. I don't like it. I know they are being kind, but I still don't like it. I used to work out for an hour every day.

Now, I can't even talk myself into walking for 15 minutes.

I used to wear classy clothes, and now I wear an elastic waist and comfortable shoes. My hair was very thick and curly. Now it's thin and scraggly. I consider myself a happy old person. I have wonderful children and grandchildren who love me.

I think about how many years I might have left, and it makes me sad. I'm 76, maybe I have 10 years, but I doubt it. Friends and acquaintances are starting to pass away.

I know not all old people feel the way I do, but the majority are going through the same things I am.

Does this old person miss being young? You bet I do!

Add what makes people feel young, such as music, fashion, or design.

## Questions:

What makes you feel young?

_____

_____

_____

Do you have fun memories of a certain activity?

_____

_____

_____

What music did you like to dance to?

_____

_____

_____

## What fashions did you wear?

_____

_____

_____

_____

_____


## Do you talk about this with your family?

_____

_____

_____

_____

_____

_____

# Fitness

"Your body is never out of shape, it is always in a shape created by how you moved up until this very moment."
— Katie Bowman
*Move Your DNA, Restore Your Health Through Natural Movement*

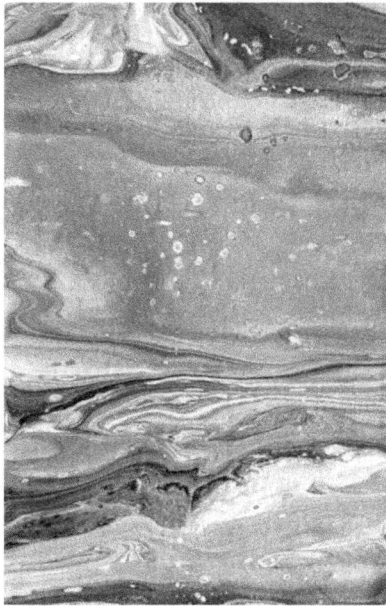

# How much exercise do older adults require?

According to the Physical Activity Guidelines for Americans, we should do at least 150 minutes of moderate exercises a week, like brisk walking or fast dancing. Being active three days a week is a good minimum. Muscle-strengthening exercises, such as weightlifting and sit-ups, are the next recommendation. This is followed by balance training to finish off the three categories.

Physical activity is great for mental and physical health. Here are some things to keep in mind when planning a routine:

- First, start slowly. Overexercising is dangerous and could cause injury.
- Begin your program slowly.
- Warm up before and cool down afterwards.
- Pay attention to your surroundings.
- Drink water before, during, and after.
- Wear appropriate clothes and shoes.
- Discuss your health conditions with your provider before proceeding.

Three questions to ask your doctor:

- Are there exercises I should avoid due to health issues?
- Is my preventive care up to date?
- What are the best exercises to keep me fit?

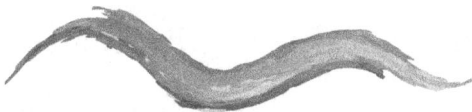

# How Does My Health Condition Affect My Ability to Exercise?

The next step: set a fitness goal.

Use the goal-setting worksheet in this chapter.

1. Write down your short-term fitness goals.

A couple of examples might be: Tomorrow, I will find out about fitness classes in my area. In the next week, I will have the shoes I need for exercising.

# Goal Setting Worksheet

1. Write down your short-term fitness goals.

_____

_____

_____

_____

_____

_____

_____

_____

_____

_____

_____

_____

_____

_____

2. Write down long-term goals.

For example: By next year, I will swim one mile three times a week. In six months, I will have my blood pressure under control.

For some people, writing a plan helps them get started and stay on target. Even if you have to break up your routine, you can make a plan, write it down, and begin again.

These suggestions are provided by the NIH National Institute on Aging, where scientists regularly review the contract to make certain it is correct and up-to-date.

## 2. Write down your long-term fitness goals

_____

_____

_____

_____

_____

_____

_____

_____

_____

_____

_____

_____

_____

_____

_____

# Stay Fit/Don't Fall

When I moved to a new home a few years ago, I needed to seek a new physician and medical team. A friend who lived near my new house suggested a local doctor, and I made an appointment.

I brought in my records, and he carefully reviewed my medical history. Then came the big lecture.

The doctor proceeded to give me a half-hour lecture on the danger of falling and how important it is to have a safe environment and to build up strength, balance, and posture to keep my body in the best condition possible.

I started working with a physical therapist in all three areas. As I look back at photos from a year and a half ago, I can say I am walking more confidently, standing straighter, and more easily adjusting for balance on uneven surfaces.

He has helped me recover from two surgeries, and I am hoping to return to regular fitness classes soon as well. I am looking forward to returning to my yoga class to work more on flexibility, balance, and strength.

Finding a way to stay fit is important as we gain the gift of extra years. Staying active and strong helps us live a more comfortable and satisfying life every day. One key is to find something you like to do that will call to you daily.

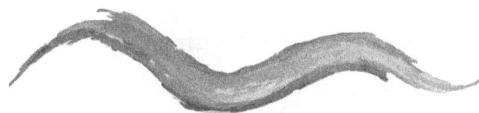

# Reliable Exercise Advice

I have friends who love to swim every day, ride a bicycle, play tennis, walk miles, or prepare to run marathons.

There are water aerobics classes for non-swimmers who want to protect their joints and still get good exercise. I recently heard some friends talking about taking up pickleball. I also know about people who have balance problems doing a yoga class where all movements are done while sitting in a chair.

Whatever you choose, it should be something that is appropriate for your level of physical fitness, safe for you to participate in, and have the flexibility to increase the challenge as you get stronger and more able to complete the workout at each stage.

# Falls

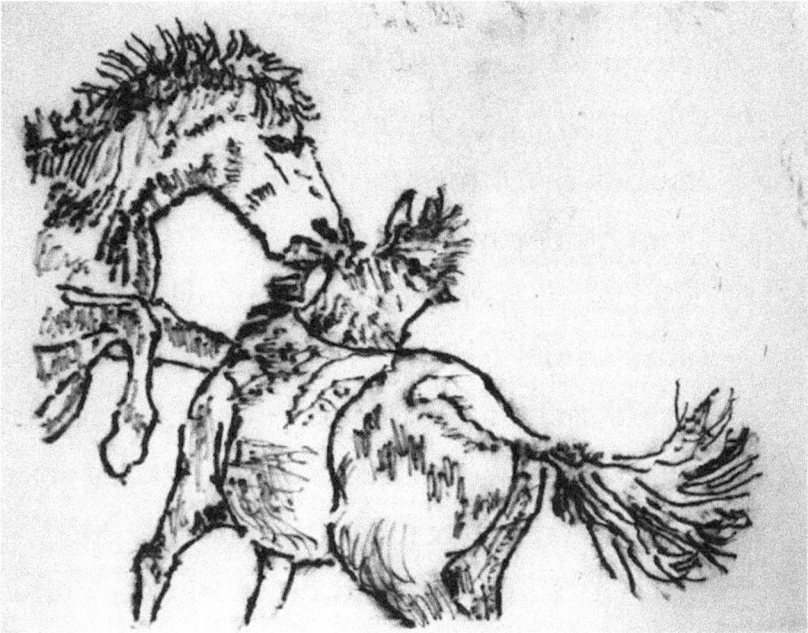

"Falls don't 'just happen' and people don't fall because they get older."
— National Institute of Health (NIH)
Senior Website

- One out of four older adults fall each year.
- As a result of falls, every 11 seconds, an older adult is treated in the emergency room. Every 19 minutes, an older adult dies.
- Falls are the leading cause of fatal and nonfatal injuries among older adults, causing hip fractures, head trauma, and death.
- Older adults are hospitalized for fall-related injuries five times more often than injuries from other causes.
- The nation spends $50 billion a year treating older adults for the effects of falls, 75% of which is paid for by Medicare and Medicaid. If fall rates are not reduced, direct treatment costs are projected to reach $101 billion by 2030.
- Fear of falling can lead older adults to limit their activities, which can result in more falls, further physical decline, depression, and social isolation.

# I Woke Up

I woke up and called a few friends and family, as I always do. Each one sounded strange to me—not at all as they usually do.

"Susan, you sounded so good," they said. Why were they saying it in a strange way? I started asking questions. My friend Judy and my cousin Kathryn said they had seen me, but I had no recollection of seeing them.

So, what did I learn?

I had another knee replacement operation that was really needed at age 80 and didn't wake up. Most people, including doctors and family, thought I was a goner.

I heard that there was an argument among family members and another between caregivers on whether to pull the plug as I was in a two-week induced coma from which half of the people believed I would never recover, and the others felt I deserved to allow my body to recover or not.

I had no recollection of the visitors or the battles. When I asked why they asked the strange question, no one gave me an explanation. I was really confused.

Generally, most of the visitors thought I would not survive and didn't know what to say when I woke up and phoned them.

I learned that my daughter thought my will was to be let go and brought my nurse up to the hospital ethics board since the nurse did not agree with her. I'm sure she didn't realize she could be destroying a career by such an action.

As it turned out, I unexpectedly woke up.

I have seen photos of myself in the coma, and it helped me to realize what caused the battle. I didn't look very alive.

# Bionic Me

Arthritis, a leading cause of disability, attacks over half of 60-year-olds in the world. But the good news is, it's something we can often overcome.

Arthritis runs in my family, so even though I have kept active and worked out regularly, my knees were bone on bone when I saw the doctor in mid-2021. The left knee was so bad I could hardly walk. The right one was also bone-on-bone but wasn't bothering me at all.

I needed a full knee replacement. The procedure was to be robotic-assisted surgery. I was told this advancement in pre-op imaging, and intra-operation navigation improves the accuracy of implant placement in addition to preserving soft tissue.

I have been pleasantly surprised by the speed at which I am recovering from the surgery and getting my mobility back. I can't wait to get back to yoga class.

My extraordinary physical therapist, Kevin Anderson, helped me prepare for surgery by making certain my leg muscles were strong. He then worked diligently to help me get my function back. I can walk again without pain, a modern miracle.

Knees, hips, and shoulders can all be replaced, and surgeries continue to get more refined and successful.

It is amazing to me that after a few short months, I can get back to my workout routine, one of the important functions of living a long life. After my knee replacement, I felt a new freedom of motion that opened the world to me. Instead of feeling old and out of the loop, I am feeling hopeful, younger, and capable of being much more active.

I recall my mother-in-law, Ann Cohn, having hip replacement surgery at the age of 90 and driving three weeks later. We have reached an era where the bionic character from television is no longer a myth. With the advances in surgery, mine was outpatient this time. I arrived at a surgi-center in the morning and was home before dinner.

The advancements in joint replacements have come a long way. When patients with arthritic hips and knees no longer respond to conservative care such as medication and physical therapy, orthopedic surgeons have the ability to replace those joints. Surgeons can often relieve pain and restore function, with great attention to safety and accuracy in order to minimize complications.

Doctors tell us that both hip and knee replacements are among the most successful and satisfying procedures for patients.

# What If What If Happens?

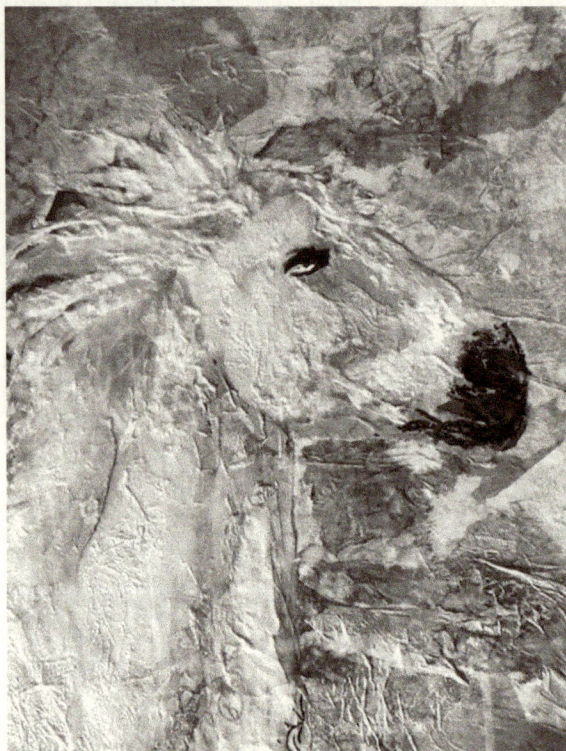

"As soon as you feel too old to do a thing, do it."

— Margeret Deland

After losing my husband to a combination of heart disease and prostate cancer, I threw myself into writing and painting. It helped me examine the long life we had together and begin to figure out how I was going to go on with life as a single person after all these years.

I wrote a book called *The Art of the Mentor* and published it within a few months. Then, I prepared a very large exhibit for the LA Art Show. The first show was postponed several months due to pandemic issues, so I did one in July and another the following January. The results of the second show were far more successful than the first, so I decided to prepare for a third the following February in 2023.

After a long week of setting up for show number two, working the show, and tearing everything down, I checked out of the downtown hotel where I had been staying all week and came home. I was tired but felt good about the week. When I stepped into my shower, it felt wonderful. That feeling is the last that I remembered when I came too, bleeding and in pain, a few minutes later.

I called out for my husband for the first time since his death. Then I quickly realized he was not there, and I was on the floor bleeding, home alone. I decided I had better get to a phone, so I crawled out of the shower to my bed and started pushing buttons on my phone. A wonderful woman who had worked the show with me answered, and I told her what was going on; she sent someone to me. The next button had my son's number on it. He came quickly and called 911. The paramedics checked me over, stabilized my neck, and rushed me to the closest hospital emergency room.

I was in the hospital for a week with 14 stitches in the gash in my head and a hard brace to stabilize my neck, which was broken in three places. That began months of rehab, not feeling like myself, and not being able to think and work as I usually do. Everything stopped. I stopped. I didn't remember a time in my life when I couldn't get started. I had no energy and no interest in completing all the projects in my studio that were waiting for attention.

I came home with a 24/7 caregiver for six weeks. I couldn't bathe by myself, change the brace, or even prepare a little something to eat. Who is this woman? I asked myself. I didn't recognize her. Where was the woman who always had multiple projects going on at once?

And it went on and on and on, week after week, month after month.

I couldn't drive, as I couldn't turn my head, so I was dependent on others for everything.

Endless, endless, endless.

Impatient, impatient, impatient and endlessly unproductive.

Have you had a time when you didn't feel like yourself? How did it make you feel?

_____

_____

_____

What did you do?

_____

_____

_____

Did you overcome the feeling? How long did it take?

_____

_____

_____

# Facing the Challenges

I must admit that as we age, we often face the possibility of a challenging or even fatal medical diagnosis. How would you face these options?

I have been challenged with thyroid cancer and breast cancer, as well as a dangerously broken neck. Each has its complications and decisions created by the diagnosis. I often see a medical diagnosis as a personal challenge to overcome, even though overcoming it is typically, at the least, an inconvenience and, at most, an opportunity to make decisions on how to live with whatever time you have and, in some cases, how long to live while doing it.

In addition, it is urgent as we age to do whatever is necessary not to fall. Falling leads to death in a large percentage of older people. The last time I moved and changed doctors, the new doctor, Dr. Mustafa Rahimi, actually took a half an hour to give me a lecture on this subject and how important it is. Within two years of the move, however, I had a mild case of Covid-19, which was what caused me to pass out in the shower.

So, with all this in mind, can you think of some things you can control/do to avoid or get through the physical challenges that will certainly come?

Here are some things to consider:

- What can you do to make your home a safer place?
- What can you do to make yourself stronger and safer in your environment?
- How can you legally prepare for various challenges?
- How can you prepare to avoid or overcome the physical challenges you or a loved one may face?

- Have you written down your wishes in an advanced directive for how you want to give people the information they need to make decisions for you in accordance with your wishes?

Here are a few tips:

- Put up safety bars in the bathroom.
- Use walking devices when told to do so by your doctor and/or therapist.
- Get out of bed and move as much as directed by your doctor and/or therapist.
- Meditate daily.
- Practice physical exercises daily: walk, do yoga, lift light weights, and learn exercises for good posture and stability.
- For those of you who are healthy, take steps to stay that way: stay active, eat well, stay involved with people, keep working, or volunteer your time to do something meaningful for others.

# Sex

"Women over sixty are still doing it-it being whatever turns them on, from doing humanitarian work to buying a dildo, from climbing Machu Picchu to having the best orgasms of their lives...Women of all ages, stand up! Follow your passions! Fall in love! Get laid!"

— **Deirdre Fishel Still Doing It: The Intimate Lives of Woman over Sixty.**

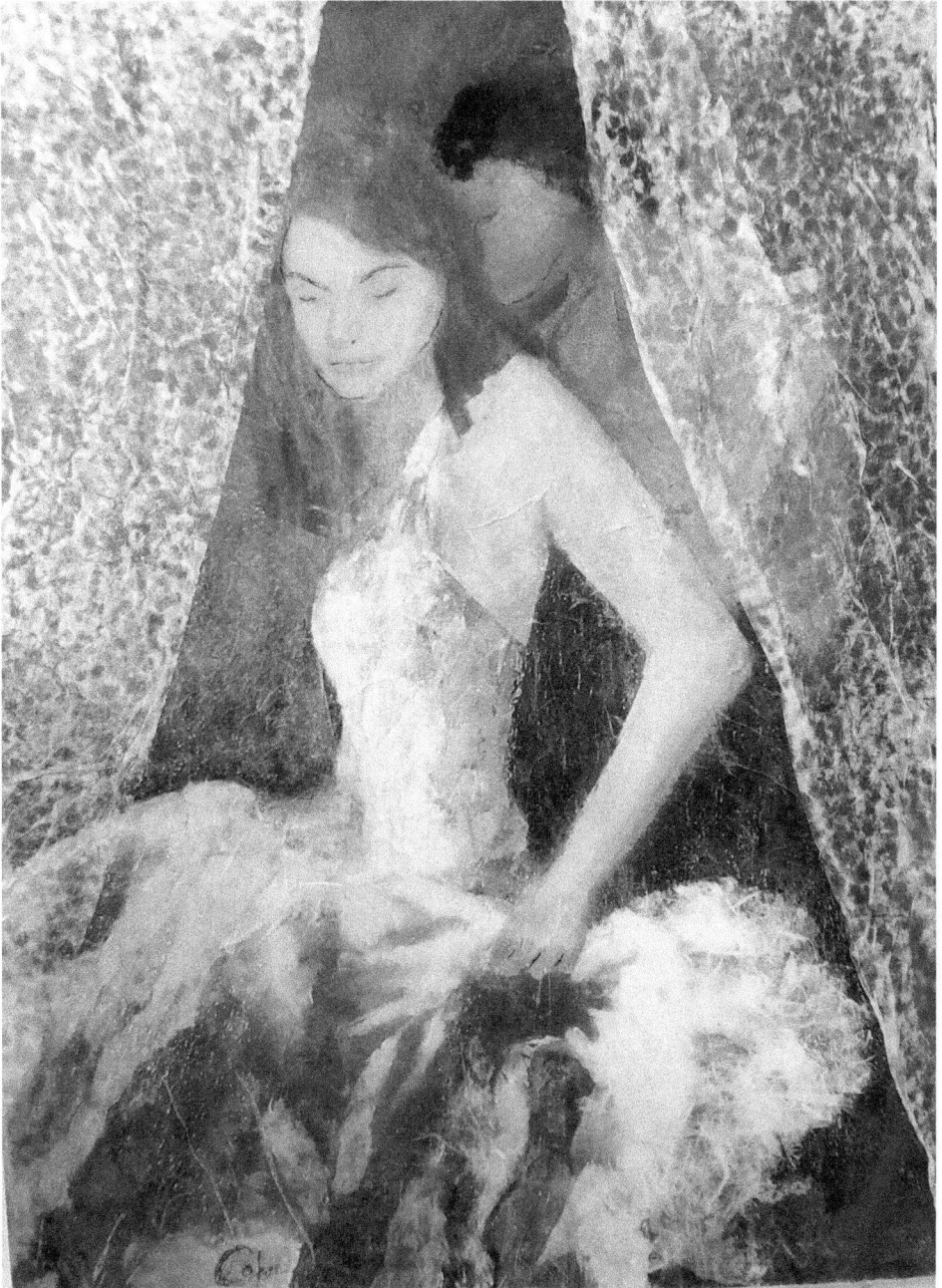

# A Fulfilling Sex Life

Despite what adult children would like to think, older adults are sexually active, according to Lindsay Wilson, MD, MPH, a geriatrician with UNC. Wilson specializes in the diagnosis and treatment of diseases in older adults and educates medical students about senior sexuality.

"People who have sex when they are older tell you it's more creative," asserts Wilson. "There is more touching. It's kind of the beauty of being older; people are more open and receptive."

Wilson enjoys advising her patients in this area as she explains that, just as with younger people, some older adults have strong sex drives and others don't. Whatever way each person feels is valid and healthy. It's unique to each person.

"For some, having sex can be a boost to emotional health and self-esteem," she says. "It might make you feel better about yourself and your body. It can be very affirming to have someone interested in you in that way. It can be a way to build connection and intimacy with a partner."

Wilson says that sex has physical benefits, as moving your body is important, and sex counts as that. One of the advantages for women is the strengthening of vaginal tissue and pelvic floor muscles.

Bodies change, and often, older couples are dealing with issues such as erectile dysfunction and dryness due to hormonal changes. Doctors can prescribe oral medications for the first and topical creams for the other. Wilson also suggests her patients seek out solutions to problems on the internet.

"Ask your doctor if your heart is healthy enough for sex," Dr. Wilson suggests as a warning.

In addition, she recommends not adding alcohol as an additional stressor. If her patient is able to walk up the steps, she takes that as a good sign. Another possible stressor for heart patients is a first-time experience with a new person, which might be problematic.

She suggests you use condoms to avoid STDs, and as for lubricants, her recommendation is for water-based ones, as oil-based lubricants can break through a condom.

"If sex is important to you, don't hesitate to talk to your partner and your doctor," she concludes. "It can be a really healthy and enjoyable part of growing older."

"All passions exaggerate; it is because they exaggerate that they are passions."
— **Sebastien-Roch Nicolas de Chamfort**

# Sexuality

After the loss of my husband of 57 years, I joined a group of grieving spouses. One of the many topics we discussed in our Covid Zoom group every week was missing the physical presence of the lost partner. No matter what our age or stage of life, most of us craved the physical closeness we had in our marriage, the ongoing comfort of touch and feel.

The National Institute on Aging says that sexuality, if you are in a relationship, is often a delicate balance of emotional and physical issues. How each person feels may affect not only what they are able to do but what they want to do.

Many older couples find greater satisfaction in their sex lives than they did when they were younger. Often, they have fewer distractions, more time, privacy, no worries about getting pregnant, possibly greater intimacy with a life-long partner, or the confidence of life experience in building new relationships later in life.

Older couples do face the same daily stressors as others. In addition, there may be added issues due to illness and life changes that can lead to difficulties. On the other hand, many of us find that it becomes easier to be clear about what we want and need as we get older. We may find it easier to talk openly with our partners, leading to more cooperation and satisfaction, even given the possibilities of limitations. Many things that cause sexual problems in older adults can be helped.

1. If you have a long-term partner, take the time to enjoy each other as well as understand the physical changes that may exist.

2. Your doctor is available to discuss these issues. She or he may be able to suggest solutions. For example, a good water-based lubricant.

3. There are medical remedies available for both men and women to make sex more satisfying.

4. In addition, adjustments to physical limitations while still finding satisfying physical contact is an option many people choose. If you are in a relationship, you and your partner may discover new ways to be together as you get older. Talk to your partner about your needs. You may find that affection—hugging, kissing, touching, and spending time together—can be just what you need, and perhaps be a pathway to greater intimacy and sex.

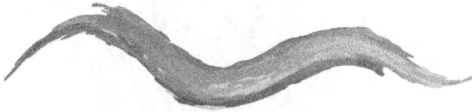

# Life After Life After Life

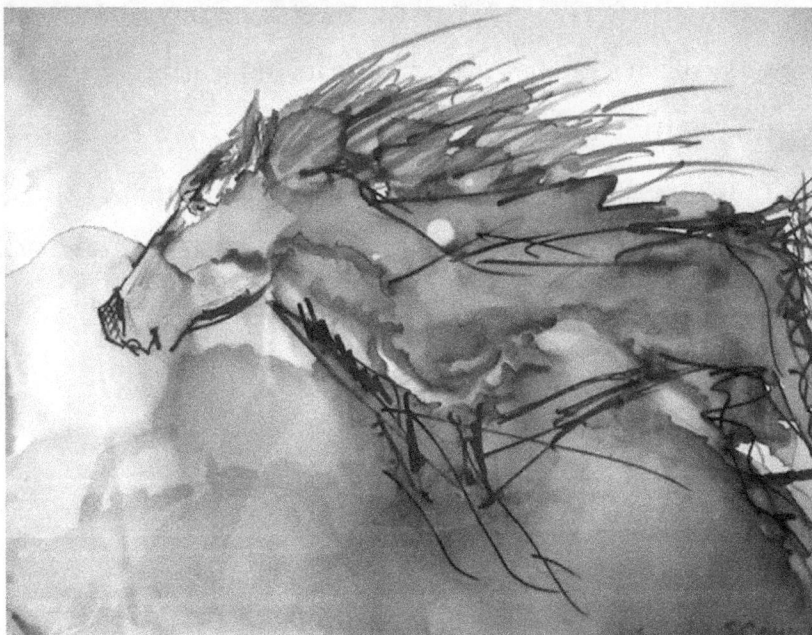

"I get up every morning with a desire to do some creative work. This desire is made of the same stuff as the sexual desire, the desire to make money or any other desire."

— Isaac Bashevis Singer

I did not expect this. I met my husband at 17. We married at 20. He died when I was 77. That is not how it was supposed to happen. I had this fantasy of the two of us walking around, holding hands, and enjoying being together well into our 90s. We both came from long-living families. Victor's mother lived to 107, and most of the women on my side of the family lived into their 90s.

So here I was, a widow. Who plans for that? It isn't actually something that you can plan for, as grief is an individual experience that moves in unpredictable fits and starts. In grief counseling, I learned that there is no grief police. Everyone has to do it in his or her own way.

My grandmother, Gretchen, was widowed fairly young. She worked hard, ran a business, parented her two children, and remained single for the rest of her life. She was my role model.

So after my husband died and I met a very kind, smart, interested man who was my age and with whom I had a lot in common, I did not expect it would move into a relationship. After all, my grandmother stayed single after my grandfather died.

Those of you who know me know that that isn't what happened.

I was used to being in a relationship with another adult, and when the opportunity arose, I said yes to an adult relationship. It was quite different from a lifelong relationship but satisfying in many ways. I felt grateful for the possibility of exploring another totally different relationship. It lasted two years.

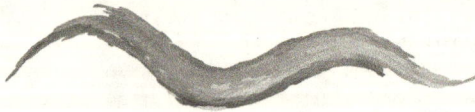

# Who, Me?

## Learn a New Way to Communicate? At My Age?

After my husband Victor retired early due to ill health, he began to look for volunteer opportunities. He had been working in the area of computers for many years, and with the advent of the personal computer, he believed he had a calling. He believed that as one aged, there was a chance of becoming isolated.

He decided he wanted to teach as many older adults as possible to use the internet. His belief was that it would eliminate loneliness if we could stay in touch with our children and grandchildren on a regular basis online, even if family wasn't nearby.

I don't have a count of the hundreds of people he shared his expertise with during those years, but it was very satisfying to him.

# Myths
## Stereotypes About Aging (That Aren't True)

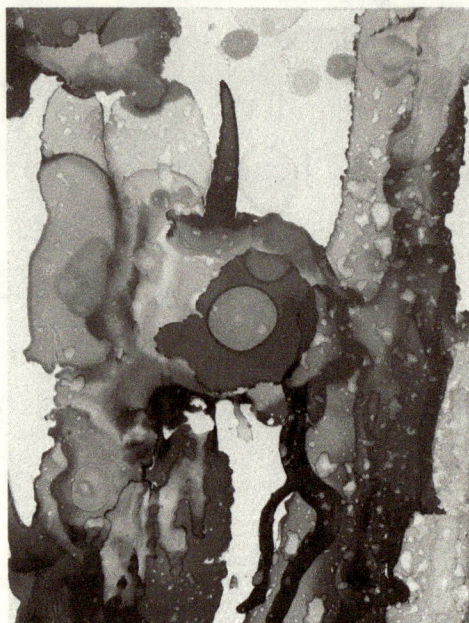

"If there's one thing I've learned in my years on this planet, it's that the happiest and fulfilled people are those who devoted themselves to something bigger and more profound than merely their own self-interest."
— John Glenn

*R*esearch has linked negative perceptions of aging in people over the age of 50 with an average 7.5-year decrease in lifespan [source: Peri].

That link could have a huge impact on our population. In 2010, people over the age of 65 comprised some 13 percent of the U.S. population. That's about 40 million Americans, a number that was expected to increase to 55 million by 2020 and the number of people aged 85 and older will increase from 5.7 million over the same period of time [source: Administration on Aging].

But it's not just the media that propagates negative stereotypes about the elderly. These blanket assumptions arise, in part, from what social scientists call the psychologist's fallacy: judging another person's state of mind based on your own experiences and perspectives [sources: Blackwell].

For example, a 40-year-old may think his 75-year-old mother will be happy to move in with his family after his father has died. She won't have to worry about keeping up a big, empty house—and you know how she loves the grandkids. His mother may see it as losing her home and independence, and being tied down with babysitting.

On the other hand, the 40-year-old and the 75-year-old might find a lot of common ground, but they'll never know until they sit down and talk about it.

When Americans think about old age, we tend to predict a slowdown, picturing ourselves in rocking chairs or perhaps in front of the television—which frequently depicts aging as bad and the elderly as ridiculous.

Members of the Tarahumara society in Mexico, on the other hand, believe that they gain strength as they age, and in their 60s, they remain able to run 100s of miles while playing a long-distance version of kickball [source: Martinez].

The lesson? The way we view the aging process may very well influence how we ourselves age.

Stereotypes:

There are six myths about old age:

1. That it's a disease, a disaster.
2. That we are mindless.
3. That we are sexless.
4. That we are useless.
5. That we are powerless.
6. That we are all alike.

"When it comes to aging, we're held to a different standard than men. Some guy said to me: 'Don't you think you're too old to sing rock n' roll?' I said: 'You better check with Mick Jagger,'" said Cher from *Fifty on Fifty: Wisdom, Inspiration, and Reflections on Women's Lives Well Lived.*

"When you get to my age, you'll really measure your success in life by how many of the people you want to have love you actually do love you... If you get to my age in life and nobody thinks well of you..., I don't care how big your bank account is, your life is a disaster. That's the ultimate test of how you have lived your life," said Warren Buffett, addressing Georgia Tech students who asked about his greatest success and failure.

# Mental and Physical Deterioration Are Inevitable in Old Age

It's true that as we age, things start to go. The loss can be staved off, however, with healthy habits. Weightlifting helps retain muscle and bone [source: Whitbourne]. Aerobic exercise and a low-fat diet improve cardiovascular health, which, in turn, can prevent certain types of dementia [source: Whitbourne].

Exercising the brain, whether by writing poetry or playing Sudoku, also helps maintain cognitive skills. As some skills diminish, others may improve to compensate. For example, concentration gets harder, and distractibility increases with age. Yet the ability to creatively use information that is acquired in the periphery during the distraction may be enhanced [source: Campbell].

However, research has shown us that believing negative stereotypes about aging can sabotage mental capacity. For instance, consider how older characters on television are often portrayed as feeble, forgetful, cranky and confused. Studies have shown a link between the amount of television watched by the aging and their own views on aging.

The more TV that older adults watch, the worse they view their own peer group and the more they buy into that stereotype, the worse they're likely to be at memory recall [source: Dominion]. In other studies, older participants who were told that they could expect to fare worse on a memory test than younger participants did indeed perform more poorly [source: Hess].

# Older People Can't Make Good Decisions About Important Issues

It's been said that age brings wisdom. Scientists would agree—except they call wisdom crystallized intelligence, by which they mean cognitive skills based on knowledge drawn from a lifetime of experience and education [source: Li et al.].

We might call it intuition or a gut feeling. This quality supplies a broader base of facts for people to base decisions on. It makes use of information that may seem unimportant to the decision at hand. Crystallized intelligence often compensates for, or complements, the critical thinking skills that typically weaken with age. As a result, older adults often make decisions that prove to be as sound as those made solely by weighing pros and cons and evaluating the reliability of sources.

Crystallized intelligence has its limits; mainly, it's overwhelmed by too much information and too many choices. But studies have shown that when the aging are removed from decisions regarding their own health care or services, they are less likely to benefit from—or even take advantage of—these services [source: Medical News Today]. This should come as no surprise. Being left out of important, personal decisions is likely to cause feelings of alienation, regardless of one's age.

# I Thought the Artist Would Be Younger

After exiting the tunnel of interactive light, sound, and art that was my installation at the 2021 LA Art Show, a member of my team asked a woman in her 20s if she would like to meet the artist.

He gestured towards me, and the woman stood absolutely still. Her face took on a pale and confused cast as she stared. At last, she spoke slowly.

"You're the artist?" she asked me…then stopped.

"I am," I replied.

Silence again. Finally, and very slowly, she responded, "I thought it was done by someone young."

"Yes," I said. "I believe that my work has no age attached to it, but I do seem to recall years ago having a similar bias regarding creative work that

I responded to as well. I assumed that if I liked a poem, for example, it must have been written by someone around my age."

A teachable moment?

An insult to her or me?

What had just happened?

What if this is a primary example of rampant ageism, the assumption that older adults are less creative or less capable of being creative?

How many times have you seen a post on the internet with an older adult singing, dancing, or playing an instrument quite well with a caption like, "awwww," "cute," or "can you believe this?"

How many years of practice and training do you think go into performances like the ones just described? Do you think making a judgement that such a performance is "cute" is an example of overt ageism?

# Why Do I Sometimes Find Old People Disgusting?

I have to laugh, NOT at the question, but it brings back a funny story that I heard.

When we were in our late 20s, my husband and I went to a restaurant, and an older man was at the next table, struggling to eat. It's like it took FOREVER for him to get the spoon to his mouth from his soup bowl, and the soup was falling everywhere. Somehow, for him, it looked like the food was farther away than it normally is from your mouth. Anyway, my husband looked at me and said, "Seriously, Christy, when I get that old, please just SHOOT me!" (So you see? You're not the ONLY one who finds old age disgusting.)

Fast forward 40 years. Naturally, my husband had become less coordinated and frail, especially after a stroke, and he called me over to help him once because he managed to get syrup ALL over the place when trying to place it on pancakes. No problem, I was there to grab a warm towel to clean him up. And while I was doing that, I said casually, "Well, I guess I better find the gun."

He said, "My gun? What for?"

I said casually, "I promised to shoot you, remember?"

We laughed so hard that the whole plate of pancakes went flying off the table!!!

So I guess my point is, even past the point of SELF-disgust, there is much to be grateful for and a whole lot of living left to do!

# Older People Don't Want or Need Close Relationships

Humans are social creatures; the need for meaningful relationships doesn't diminish with age. If older adults give off that impression, it may be because they have increasingly fewer people to relate to as they age. Friends die. Family members move away. Physical and mental impairment can make even short visits an ordeal.

Perhaps not surprisingly, then, one in three people in their 60s are chronically lonely, a condition associated with a host of illnesses from high blood pressure to Alzheimer's disease. Feelings of loneliness do drop with each decade aged afterwards—partially as people's overall satisfaction with their lives tends to rise after the age of 50 [source: Edmonson].

Ongoing social relationships reap numerous benefits. In fact, the challenge of interacting with others has been found to help maintain information-processing skills, like perceiving spatial relationships between objects [source: HealthDay News].

The more people whom an older adult can rely on in times of trouble, and the more varied these relationships, the less stress there will be in that person's life [source: Powell].

# Older People Aren't Interested in Sex or Intimacy

It's hard for some younger people to think that their parents and even their grandparents are having sex—and enjoying it, but don't take our word for it. In several comprehensive surveys, older adults described their sex lives in intimate detail.

The findings include:

- Positive sexual relationships were found to be associated with overall well-being. Whether one caused the other wasn't clear [source: Law].
- Individuals' sexual activity remained constant until about age 70. Normal changes due to aging and age-related health problems were obstacles in older age [source: University of Chicago].
- While most respondents aged 70 and over said that sex was less important as they age,

only about 35 percent said that sex is only for married people, and less than 10 percent said it's only for the young.

- Of this same group, most felt that their partners found them physically attractive. They praised their partners as loving and gentle.

- In general, women ranked sex less important than relationships and overall quality of life than men did. That may be because women are more likely to outlive their spouses, and older widows may feel less interested in starting a new intimate relationship. Also, older women outnumber older men, leaving fewer potential partners [source: Fisher].

- Most respondents hadn't talked to their doctor about sex since they were 50. Researchers think that with better information, older adults might enjoy more rewarding relationships.

# As You Get Older, You Get More Set in Your Ways

Evidence from a number of fronts has shown that older adults are more open to change than the popular image might lead you to believe. For example, the number of people ages 65 and older who use Twitter nearly doubled from 2009 to 2010 [source: Madden]. And more unmarried older couples are choosing cohabitation over marriage compared to previous generations, even compared to today's younger couples.

On a deeper level, older people tend to have high levels of mental resilience, which is the ability to accept and rebound from adversity [source: Berk]. Being resilient often means giving up self-defeating habits and attitudes, whether it's smoking or self-pity, and adopting new ones. Also, the happiest older adults say that their perspective changed as they realized that their lives were coming to a close. The concerns of their younger days faded, and they began focusing on the satisfaction of living in the moment [source: Graham].

# Older People Want to Die

Like decision-making, this is another stereotype that can't be easily labeled true or false. Older adults are more accepting of death when they feel some sense of control over it. Generally, they want to ensure a "happy" death in a comforting environment, knowing that they're loved and free of unnecessary pain.

To one person, that's achieved by making out a living will that specifies the type of end-of-life medical treatment he or she wants. To another, that peace of mind comes from having the option of physician-assisted suicide. But it wouldn't be fair to say that either person wants to die.

To complicate matters, impressions can be deceiving. For instance, older people may talk more about dying as it becomes more and more of a reality. Also, grief and depression caused by chronic illness or the loss of a spouse can certainly make death seem more welcome.

# Older People Aren't Interested in the Outside World

Not even close to the stereotypical image of being technophobic or sedentary TV watchers, today's adults are taking advantage of ways to stay mentally and physically engaged. One example is, in 2010 alone, almost 100,000 people explored international culture through Elderhostel, an organization that offers enriching travel and educational programs for older adults throughout the world [source: Elderhostel].

Plus, many seniors take part in continuing education programs: The Osher Lifelong Learning Institutes, a network of educational programs designed for learners ages 50 and up, has locations on close to 120 campuses throughout the United States [source: Bernard Osher Foundation].

In fact, a growing number of retirement communities are built near colleges and universities, using access to on-campus classes and enrichment events as a selling point. Some of the facilities give preference to alumni and former professors, who give lectures on the community grounds.

## Science Has Answered All Our Questions About Aging

It's worth stating that there's a lot we still don't know about old age and the aging process. As people live longer than ever before, science is accruing more data regarding the oldest age group, those aged 85 and up. It's a good thing as well because 90-year-olds are the fastest-growing age group of the U.S. population [source: U.S. Census].

This data could answer a number of questions. For example, if we can slow the development of Alzheimer's disease in a 70-year-old, will the benefits last when that person is 85 or 95? How will the average dietary habits of today's 40-year-olds impact them 40 years down the road?

While the answers to those questions are still pending, perhaps the wisest attitude regarding aging and older adults comes in these words, supposedly given to us by Mark Twain: "Age is an issue of mind over matter. If you don't mind, it doesn't matter."

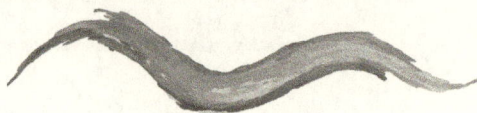

# Inspiration: The Stones

I attended a Rolling Stones concert in mid-2021 in Los Angeles at the new football stadium. Tens of thousands of people were there and yet I felt involved and part of the experience the whole time. They put on an outstanding show, but beyond that, there was a realization that Mick Jagger and I are the same age, which gave it enhanced meaning for me.

As the frontman of the group, Jagger never stops moving. He runs, jumps, skips, waves, and gestures throughout the show without a break, changing costumes several times in the process. It made me want to stand, sing along, and dance, which I did joyfully.

So, Jagger became the role model for so many of us in the audience. I took some photographs of people walking out after the concert. The fun of the photos is the variety of ages of the attendees, including quite a few couples and singles that appeared to be in my age range with lots of grey hair and imperfect bodies dancing in the aisles and happily walking toward parking lots.

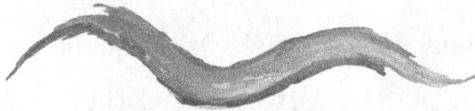

# Older People Contribute to Society

People often treat older adults like antique autos. The assumption is you can take them for a Sunday drive in the park, but you wouldn't try to get any real work out of them. In other words, they were useful in their prime but no longer.

This is not based on truth. With years of personal skills and professional expertise, older adults are a highly valued volunteer force. Senior Corps, for example, boasts 500,000 members ages 55 and up, meeting community needs that range from mailing newsletters for nonprofits to fostering hard-to-place children [source: Senior Corps].

And older adults who participate in Mentor: The National Mentoring Partnerships, advise and encourage high school students in navigating the challenges of school, relationships, and career planning.

Older workers can be assets to businesses, too. In surveys, employers have reported that older workers are more reliable and have a stronger work ethic than younger workers. They also take fewer sick days.

Some people blaze history-making trails in later life. American primitivist painter Anna Mary "Grandma" Moses took up art at the age of 75 when arthritis made embroidery too difficult. One of her paintings sold for $1.2 million in 2006. Similarly, Mary Harris "Mother" Jones hit her stride as a worker's rights activist when she was in her 60s, earning her the title of "the most dangerous woman in America" [source: AFL-CIO].

# Money

"The longer I live, the more beautiful
life becomes."
— Frank Lloyd Wright

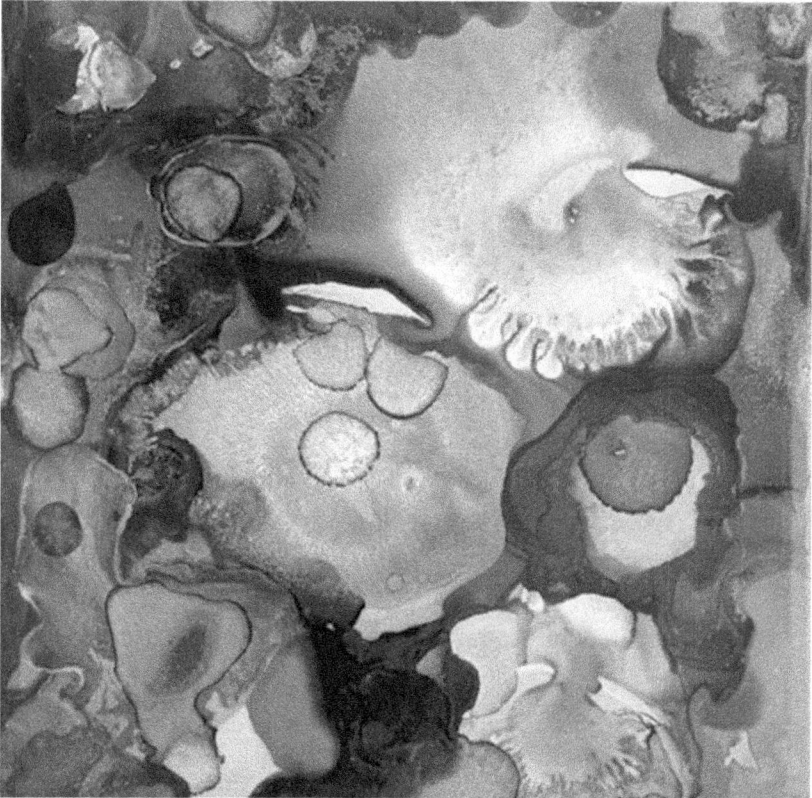

# How to Make Money Last

How many more years do you have to live?

28 percent of Americans 50 and older underestimate their life expectancy by five years or more, according to the Society of Actuaries.

The downside of this pessimistic view is the possibility that one might run out of money. When underestimating longevity, money managers indicate that it can lead to putting away too little savings or retiring too early before reaching a level of financial stability for the potential life span of the saver.

Many tools are available to help project a lifespan for budgeting your assets for retirement. If you search online for a life-expectancy calculator, you can try several to get an idea of how to project your life span.

# Make a Plan

Whatever number you come up with, add a few years for good measure and safety to ensure your resources will last for your lifetime. In fact, a Chicago financial planner, Donald Duncan, has been quoted as saying that many of his clients have financial plans that run through age 100.

After the exercise of projecting a possible life span, you can make a spending plan for that period of time. If you come up short on covering the expenses found in your initial projections, it's time to cut back. For many Americans, that means giving your children more of your time and less of your money.

In a recent poll, it turns out that nearly 80% of parents who helped their offspring during the pandemic said they gave money they would have otherwise used to improve their own financial situation.

# Review Health Coverage Regularly

Don't put your Medicare enrollment on autopilot. Each year, as your needs change, you can reevaluate your budget and projected healthcare needs for the coming year and reallocate the funds in a way that works with your financial needs. Medicare has an Extra Help program, which could be used to reduce costs considerably.

# Identify Ways to Cover Basic Needs

Most retirees like to know they can cover basic needs like food and housing with monthly income, no matter what happens. The social security payment comes first. Does it cover these basics?

Do you have other income, such as a rental property, that brings in a regular amount of money each month? Do you have a part-time job or hobby that brings in some monthly income? If you own a home, have you looked into a reverse mortgage? Though they are complicated and have fees, there are counseling agencies available to assist the borrower.

Another possibility is a longevity annuity that, when purchased, pays the borrower a monthly sum for life that can create needed income.

## Look for Community Resources Set Up to Assist Seniors

Many communities offer financial counseling, low-cost loans, and other help. Check resources in your town for low to no-cost services.

# Watch Out for Scams

Scams have increased during the pandemic, according to the FBI. Keep your resources safe by gathering a group of friends and family to advise you about any investment opportunity or request for emergency funds.

A very smart and aware couple that I know was taken in by a caller who claimed their grandson was in trouble in another country and needed money immediately. They had wired thousands of dollars before discovering their grandson was safely home in bed.

And finally, give someone you trust power of attorney to make financial decisions on your behalf in case you become incapacitated.

# Telling Your Story

"It's a wrong idea that a master is a finished person. Masters are very faulty; they haven't learned everything and they know it."

— Robert Henri

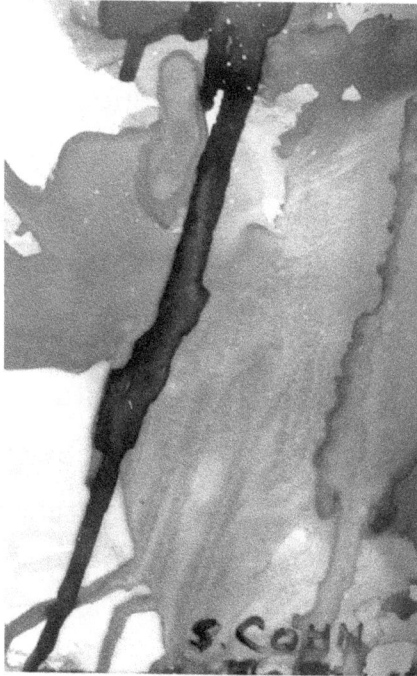

Nobody knows the details of your life but you. Often, your children and grandchildren have questions about family history and traditions that don't get asked until it is too late to get answers.

If each of us tries to gather photos and record stories about our childhood, our siblings, our parents, and our grandparents, the questions will be answered without asking.

Years ago, my mother reached up into her closet and handed me a handwritten manuscript by my grandmother's uncle. It included photos of his parents and siblings, along with where they lived and where they were educated. It is a treasure and led to having information for a family tree going back many generations, plus records of interests and expertise of those that came before us. Because I have it, when a cousin is looking for information, they often contact me. I also contact cousins who have other pieces of the family history puzzle.

Some years ago, I wrote a column in the Jewish Newspaper in the Coachella Valley (Palm Springs area) about finding information about family history. I told a story in each issue about an ancestor or cousin or family lore and how I found out about it. The column attracted a lot of questions from readers asking how to follow and record family information.

Even if you have not begun to intentionally find and write down family stories, you can begin by writing down memories of how holidays were spent when you were a child, what the most memorable times you spent with your grandparents were, or your favorite activities from your childhood. This is a great opportunity to explore your family history and make sure your story is remembered for decades to come.

Stories that are not passed down from one generation to the next will eventually be lost and forgotten. You are the only one who knows your story. Take the time and opportunity to write or record it for future generations.

In addition to writing your own memories, you can write those of parents, grandparents, aunts, and uncles by preparing questions, setting aside quiet time and finding a quiet place, using your phone to record and transcribe answers, and listening actively to be certain you are getting the details of a story.

To begin these conversations, it is beneficial to view old family photos together and use open-ended questions like, "What do you remember about your grandparents?"

In addition, don't forget to ask specific questions such as, "Where was your mother born?"

Some other questions you can ask when trying to assist an older relative to recall their memories so they can be preserved include:

## Is there anything you regret not asking your parents?

_____

_____

_____

_____

_____

_____

_____

_____

_____

_____

_____

What was the happiest moment of your life?

_____

_____

_____

How would you like to be remembered?

_____

_____

_____

What was school like for you as a child?

_____

_____

_____

Which new technology have you found most helpful in your life?

_____

_____

_____

Who influenced your life the most?

_____

_____

_____

Do you have a lost love?

_____

_____

_____

# Retire

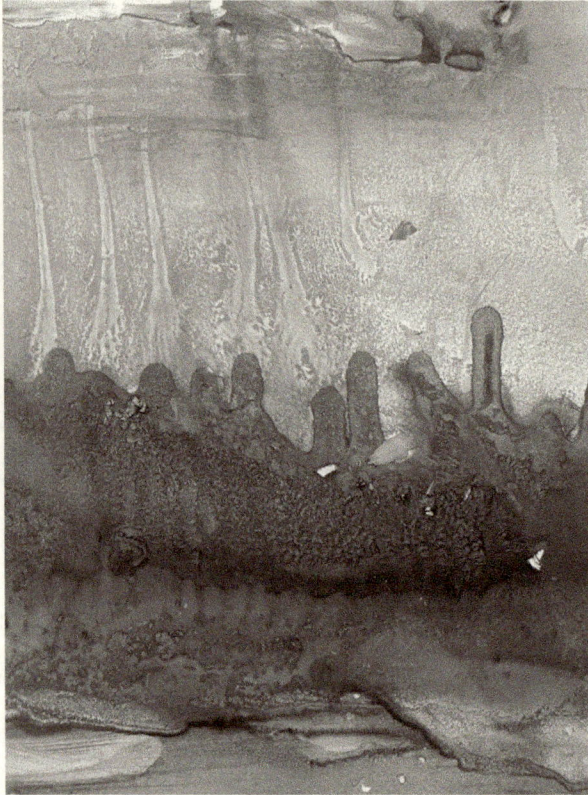

"I'm working, but there is so much still to be done! And it frightens me to think of my weight of years. But on we go, without fear or hesitation."
— Giacomo Puccini

# Ideal Age to Retire?

According to researcher Daniel Levitin, Ph.D., the ideal retirement decision is not to do it. He emphasizes that too much time spent with no purpose can lead to unhappiness.

Many employers in the USA allow older workers to modify their work schedules to be able to continue working. Laws around the world vary, with some countries requiring retirement at 60 or 65, but researchers say it's best to keep actively working either in a job or as a volunteer.

Economists use the word unretirement to describe the fact that many who retire don't like it and go back to work. It is estimated that between 25% and 40% of retirees return to the workforce after retirement.

Levitin interviewed people between the ages of 70 and 100 to gain an understanding of what helps them be satisfied with their lives. He found that all of them continued to work, giving them a sense of purpose, an active brain, and the all-important social engagement.

## Retirement Continued

We need to work together to fight for changes in the way our society sees older adults, particularly in the workforce. Corporate culture in the US tends to lean towards ageism. It is often difficult for older adults to get a job or get promoted.

Two-thirds of American workers say they have witnessed or experienced age discrimination at work. Employers who hire older workers discover that it's a smart business move. Multi-generational teams including older members tend to be more productive.

I have friends who continue to be involved in the world after retirement. They volunteer their time in various areas. There is always a need for volunteer tutors to help students increase literacy and test scores. In addition, I have friends who are museum docents and love spending their time volunteering in that capacity. There are many stimulating volunteer opportunities available.

Taking classes online is another way many of my friends expand their minds, in addition to joining book clubs, discussion groups, or volunteering in a hospital or soup kitchen.

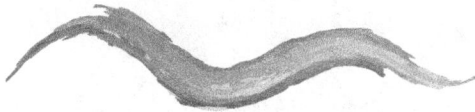

# Blue Zones

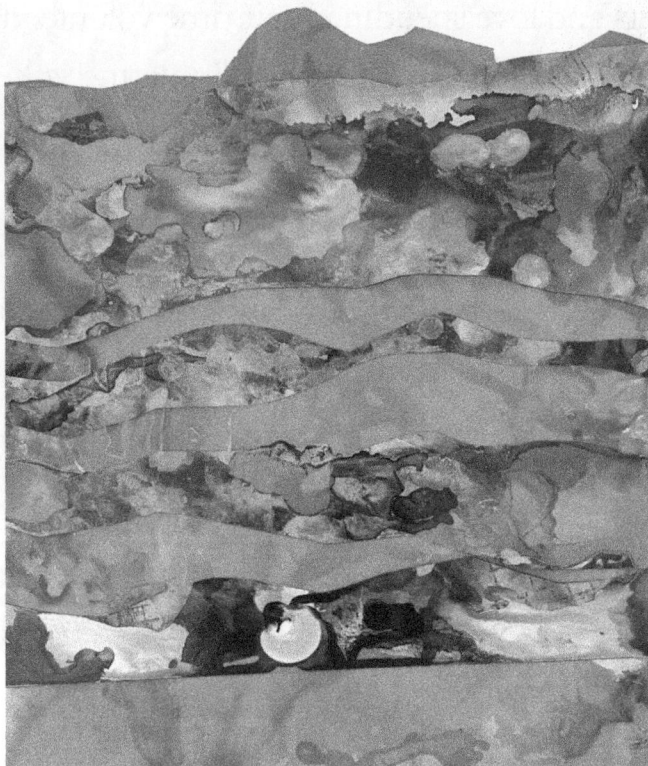

"We have a responsibility to make our lives a blessing for the planet and for the people we love, as well as for ourselves."

— Ilchi Lee

# Blue Zones

For many years, author Dan Buettner has worked to discover blue zones, which are areas of the world where residents live longer lives than those in other areas. He then studied what is different about the habits of people in those areas.

There is only one blue zone that he has identified in the USA, Loma Linda, and it is near where I live in Southern California. This community has the highest concentration of Seventh-day Adventists in the United States. Many residents from different ethnic backgrounds live 10 more years than the average American lifespan by following what's known as the biblical diet of grains, fruits, nuts, and vegetables.

At 100, Benita Welebir is chatty and observant. What is extraordinary about her longevity is that it isn't extraordinary at all in Loma Linda. She is just another old person, just like one of her neighbors who is 101 and another who is 100. After their morning exercise class, several of these friends take a walk outside.

The mother of five claims she is very energetic, that her legs are wearing out a bit, and that she has always been happy.

Loma Linda University has collected huge quantities of data from thousands of people over the years. Their faith instructs them to treat their bodies as temples: little to no meat or fish, no smoking or alcohol, plenty of exercise, and a sense of purpose.

Loma Linda Market has bin after bin of beans and grains but no meat section. The data shows that a 30-year-old Adventist man is likely to live more than seven years longer than the average white California man. For women, it was a 4.4-year difference. The differences were greater for vegetarian Adventists.

# Can You Make Your Home a Blue Zone?

Dan Buettner, who studies and writes about the blue zones, was recently featured in an issue of National Geographic, reissued in 2021.

People who live in the blue zones live longer and healthier lives, as indicated in the Loma Linda study. There is a lot more information that is worth pursuing in this issue, such as what it takes to develop a blue zone. One person or one family can start making changes at home, which can make a difference.

I will include a few tips for those who are interested, but you should check out the National Geographic issue on blue zones, which has chapter after chapter of ideas that are easy to follow.

The following are a few of its edicts:

- Make breakfast your largest meal, including protein, complex carbohydrates, and plant-based fats. Expand your idea of breakfast to include items like miso soup, beans, and corn.
- Try to eat breakfast at home. Eat with others. Say grace or have a moment of silence before eating. Plate food in the kitchen. People who eat family-style eat up to 30% more.
- Establish a family rule that everyone eats dinner together.
- Never eat standing up.
- Four foods to focus on: whole wheat bread, nuts, beans (dried or canned), and fresh fruit.
- Four foods to avoid: sugar-sweetened beverages (empty calories), too much salt or preservatives, processed meats (leads to cancer and heart disease), and packaged sweets. Ban candy and cookies from the pantry.
- Buettner suggests seeing that your diet is 95 to 100% plant-based. He says to keep favorite fruits and vegetables on hand. If fresh isn't

available, his backup is frozen. Olive oil is a substitute for butter. Then, stock up on whole grains such as oats, barley and brown rice. Grains in the blue zone tend to have less gluten.

● Research suggests that 30-year-old vegetarian Adventists will likely outlive their meat-eating counterparts by as much as eight years.

## Your ideas to try yourself:

_____

_____

_____

_____

_____

_____

_____

_____

_____

_____

_____

_____

_____

# Ethical Will

"If you are pining for youth I think it produces a stereotypical old man because you only live in memory, you live in a place that doesn't exist. Aging is an extraordinary process where you become the person you always should have been..."

— David Bowie

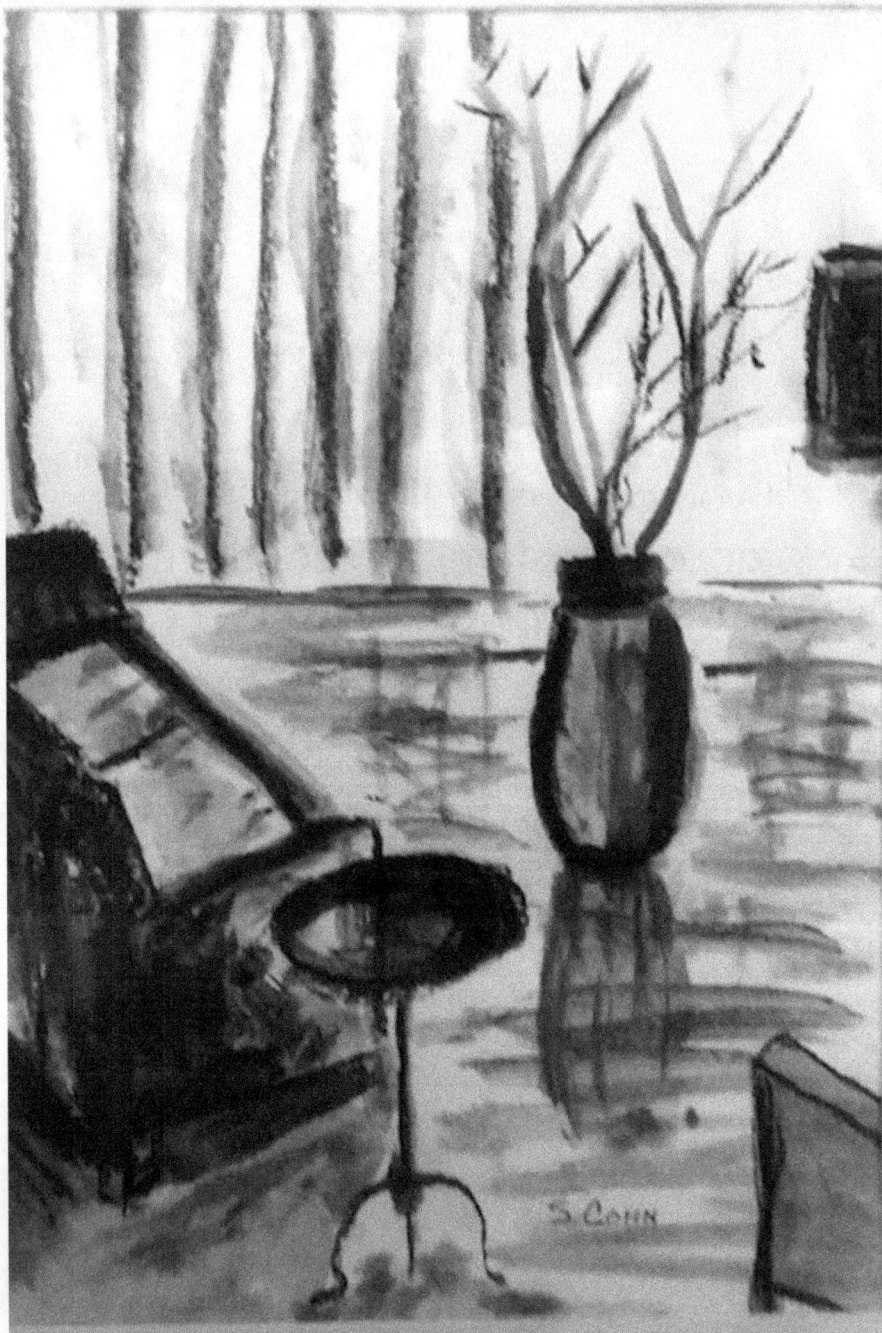

# What Is an Ethical Will and Why Do I Want One?

An ethical will is a personal document that you create to communicate your values, experiences, and life lessons to your family. It is purely voluntary and unlike a legal will as it does not discuss the distribution of assets.

The ethical will originated in ancient Jewish tradition. The original template came from Genesis 49:1 - 33. A dying Jacob gathered his sons to offer them his blessings and request that they bury him in Canaan instead of Egypt. In another biblical example in Deuteronomy 32:46 - 47, Moses instructs the Israelites to be a holy people and to teach their children.

In the medieval period, ethical wills contained directions from fathers to their children or from aged teachers to their disciples. Because they were not designed for publication, they often revealed the writer's innermost feelings and ideals.

A very early ethical will was written by Eleazar, the son of Isaac of Worms, in about 1050 CE. He exhorts those he writes to, "Think not of evil, for evil thinking leads to evil doing...purify the body, the dwelling-place of the soul...Give of all thy food a portion to God. Let God's portion be the best and give it to the poor."

Later, in the 16th through 18th centuries, they became more sophisticated.

Today, ethical wills are written by men and women of every age, ethnicity, faith, tradition, economic circumstance, and education level. The ancient ethical will was designed to transmit ethical instructions to future generations, modern heirs resist being controlled from the grave, but readily accept spiritual blessings from elders.

The content of an ethical will may be similar to a memoir or biography but is differentiated by its intention to transmit love and learning to future generations. Writing can include the following:

- family history
- cultural and spiritual values
- blessings and expressions of love
- pride in hopes and dreams for children and grandchildren
- life lessons and wisdom of life experience
- requests for forgiveness or regretted actions
- rationale for philanthropic and personal financial decisions
- stories about meaningful objects going to heirs
- clarification about and personalization of advance health directives
- requests for ways to be remembered after death

A friend was telling me that he would like to tell his grandchildren some things about his life that he thought were important regarding his beliefs and how he lived. I remembered a workshop I attended several years ago at the Alpert JCC in Long Beach,

CA. We addressed the Jewish tradition of writing an ethical will and the way to do it. It was a moving experience for all of us who attended, and we spent the day drafting our first attempt at a letter to our descendants. We learned and wrote, and at the end of the day, many of us read aloud what we had been writing all day. There were many tears and much laughter as we read the deeply meaningful documents we had created in the one-day workshop.

There is no right or wrong time of life to do this. It is always a good time to think about life lessons you have learned that you would like to pass on. You can begin as a young adult or wait to share memories and experiences that you would like to share with family after a lifetime.

## How do I begin?

Think through significant events and experiences in your life. What were the happiest and most challenging moments? What would you like your family to know about your hopes for their future? It might be a place for an apology never spoken. Or it could begin with family stories that have been passed down in the family.

There are no rules or format. It could be a letter, a scrapbook, a recording, a collage, or a PowerPoint presentation. It could just as easily be a song or a poem.

A few of the possible areas you might consider are:

- Your personal history, such as where you were born and what your family was like.
- Details about marriage proposals, divorces, and lessons learned.
- Favorite people, places, and things and why.
- Academic and professional achievements and disappointments.
- Religious and political beliefs and causes you care about.
- Values and wishes for the future.
- A mistake you made that your family could avoid.
- An experience you hope your family might have someday.

# How to Get Started

Answer the following questions to begin your thinking process:

1. What are three core values in your life?

_____

_____

_____

_____

_____

2. Identify three courageous choices you made that were driven by your personal, work, and communal values.

_____

_____

_____

_____

_____

3. Recall an experience when your values were challenged, and how you fought to uphold them.

_____

_____

_____

4. Think about the private ways you remain connected to your past.

_____

_____

_____

5. Identify a past and present moral dilemma in your life and chart the impact of making a courageous decision rather than a convenient one.

_____

_____

_____

6. Consider: what gives my life meaning?

_____

_____

_____

_____

_____

7. Consider: if I had to live my life over again, what would I do with it?

_____

_____

_____

_____

_____

# Continue Forward

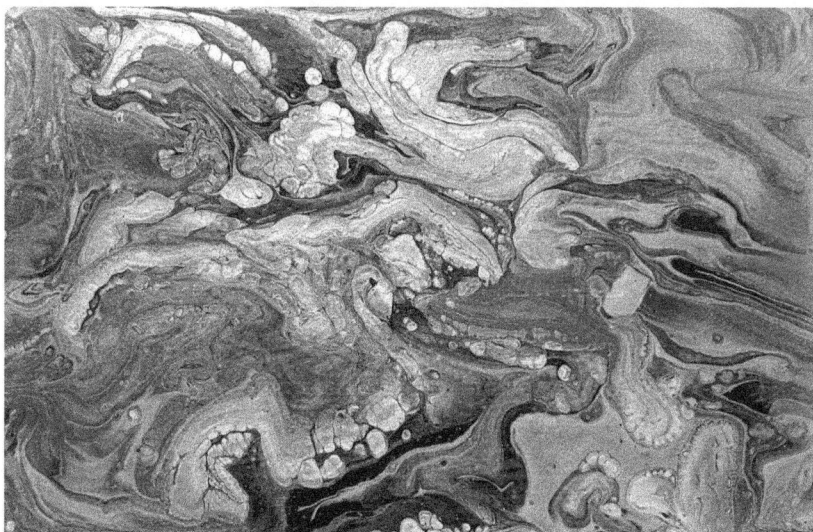

"Aging isn't a problem or disease. Aging is living."
— Ashton Applewhite

# Partial List Made Up by Program Planners and Caregivers
## for a Long Productive Life

Learn and exercise your brain regularly.

Be gentle with yourself, listen to inner voices, and do what feels best.

Get a massage, touch feels good.

Smile a lot.

Get sufficient rest.

Drink and eat in moderation.

Simplify parts of your life, one at a time.

Embrace technology and go where the internet can take you.

Keep growing as long as you are breathing.

Don't try to be everything to everyone; it is not possible.

Eliminate multitasking. Research says we do not do it well.

Meditate and/or pray daily.

Treat others with respect and dignity. It comes back to you.

Maintain muscle mass to prevent falls.

Get a pedometer and walk 5,000 to 10,000 steps a day.

Eat with friends and family.

Eat food that you like.

Laugh and cry, but laugh more.

Do not let yourself be diminished by anyone. You are you, be proud of it.

Write letters, blogs, stories, diaries, anything that gets your brain working. You are never too old for new friendships. Embrace change. Life is change. Resisting is a waste of energy.

Embrace the joys of old age when you are smarter, more experienced, and have time to do things you enjoy.

Each morning, think of five things you are grateful for before getting out of bed.

Get an annual physical checkup.

Appreciate every day.

Make your home a special place by personalizing it.

Make it a point to share joy whenever you can.

Everyone has accomplishments. Celebrate yours and others.

We can not imagine how opportunities will present themselves; we just need to be open to them.

Have someone in your life you can say anything to.

Spend time with other generations.

# Audience Members in Their 70s and 80s
## Surveyed on Their Tips for a Long, Productive Life

Develop an appropriate diet.

Get involved in meaningful, joyful, peaceful, or charitable opportunities.

Stay involved with family.

Stay involved with friends.

Give back to society.

Take care of your body: eat well, stay active, listen to doctors, and catch problems early.

Do not get stuck in the minutiae of life.

Do not forget about others—look for balance, paying attention to your own needs, but also what others need.

Hope is essential.

Hold on to joy and a positive attitude.

Eat lots of vegetables and less red meat.

Keep your mind active.

Keep your body active.

Love even through the hard times—face whatever and move forward.

Humor!

Accept life as drops of water and slowly start carving a path with new terms.

Routine is a series of actions based upon the role you are in—when our role as best friend, wife, etc.

is over, we must learn new skills, find new roles, and move forward.

Enjoy your life's work—I taught English for 40 years and loved it, married well, and just celebrated 30 years.

Get out of town often, at least annually. I am in Utah and Oregon for theater, for starters.

Have hobbies.

Collect something that gives you pleasure and reasons to keep collecting.

Have supportive family and friends.

Be nice.

Be optimistic.

Be loving.

And expect the above in return.

# What Can I Do Today?

That question is good to ask daily for keeping young and active. Is there a senior center in your community? Check it out. When I looked at the one nearby, I discovered that there was a meet and greet every Monday. This turned out to be a discussion group featuring baked goods and an open discussion each week. Before long, I met new people and looked forward to seeing them.

On Tuesday afternoons, there was a writing group. We brought our writings each week and used the opportunity to get feedback. For me, this was a favorite couple of hours of the week.

On Wednesdays, there was a fascinating lecture series. All of these were free of charge apart from a small membership fee.

Thursdays was a 'do your own craft' session for those who enjoy spending time with others while doing arts and crafts.

On Fridays, there were a variety of games.

Check out your local senior center or community center.

# Other Group Suggestions

Book clubs
Grief counselling
Art groups
Singing groups

Learn something new—challenge yourself.

# Do you have regular activities you look forward to?

_____

_____

_____

_____

_____

_____

_____

_____

_____

_____

_____

_____

_____

_____

_____

# Preparation for Retirement Checklist

**A**nother thing you can do today is prepare for retirement.

What do you want or expect your life to look like when you retire?

Get your finances in order. How much income do you need to retire? How much money will be available to you monthly, and from what sources? Do you need to reduce your current spending to provide income for more years than you had originally expected?

What do you have to do to ensure you have enough? What circumstances might have to be considered? We have lived through inflation, recession, and a pandemic...how would you handle each of these situations if they occurred during your retirement years?

How are you taking care of your body, considering our aging population? Do you do at least 150 minutes of physical activity a week? If not, what activity could you add that you would enjoy?

Do you get regular medical check-ups? Do you have a preventive healthcare routine?

Do you have a social network? Family? Friends? People with common interests who gather regularly to enjoy this shared activity?

Do you make plans to do things you enjoy? A spa day? A concert? What activity do you most enjoy doing?

Have you made plans to travel? It keeps us young to visit places we have always wanted to go. Do you like to fly? Cruise? Camp?

Do you volunteer your time? Are you doing something that helps others?

Do you have one or more outlets that you want to pursue?

Do you have a "bucket list" of places you want to go or things you want to pursue?

In conclusion don't spend these extra years in front of the television. Take inspiration from the long-livers who have already made it past the average age, and prepare for the extra years that may be in your future.

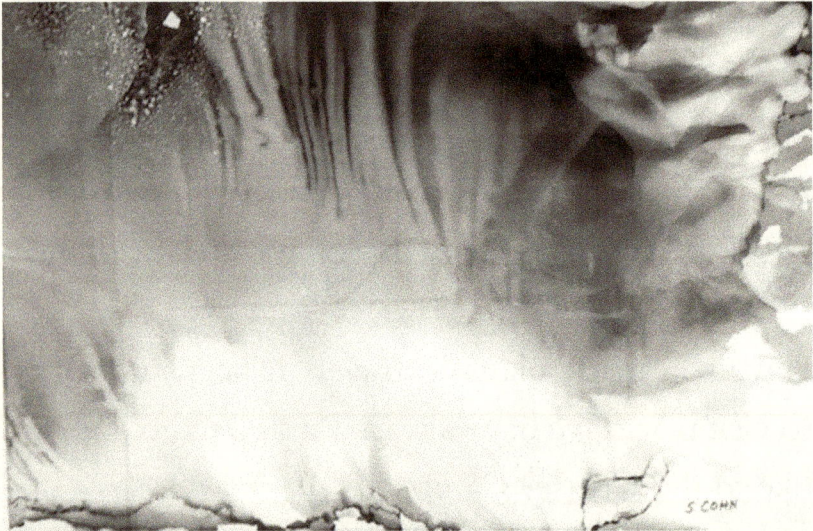

Atmosphere

# About the Author

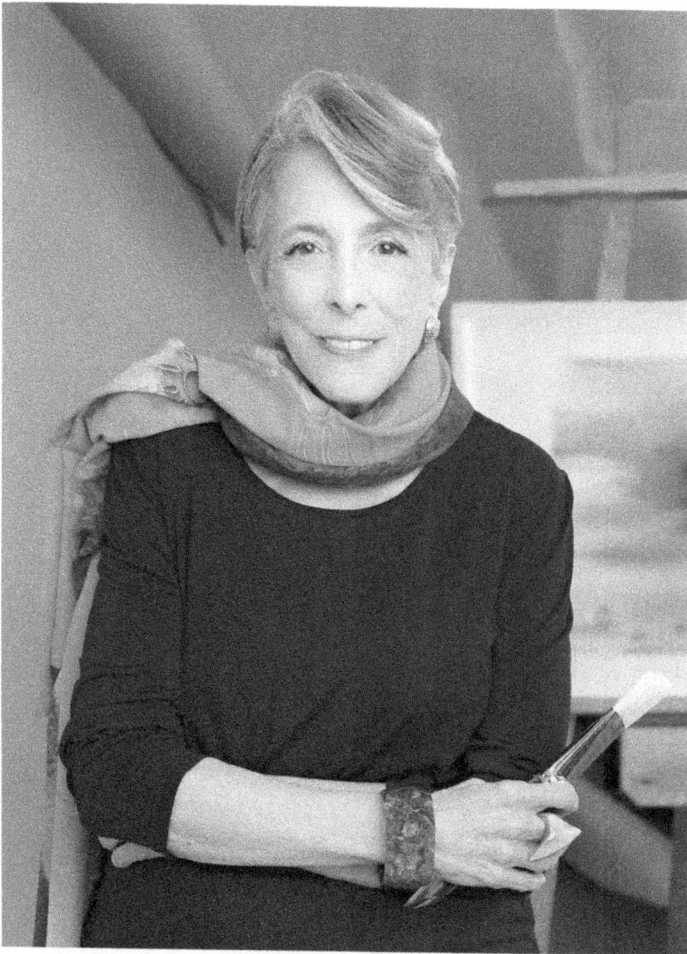

Susan Soffer Cohn grew up in a huge family of parents, grandparents, aunts, uncles, and cousins, all of whom shared their interests and supported the other members of the family in whatever they pursued. Because of this, her early childhood involved a lot of mentoring from her many, many close relatives. An example of the size of her family is that 500 people were invited to her wedding, and almost all were close relatives.

One grandmother took her to see historic houses, the other took her to work, so she learned about business. An aunt introduced her to classical music and a great aunt took her to the opera and the theater.

Focusing on experimental art, her work has been exhibited throughout the United States and Europe and in Australia. Her work has also been featured in Professional Artist Magazine in the USA and Australian Artist Magazine.

Susan began painting at 50 and studied with carefully chosen mentors who were talented artists as well as master teachers. She currently lives in the Los Angeles South Bay area. She has painted daily for over 20 years.

As Susan discovered her fulfilling life as an artist, she now dreams of helping the people she meets to find out what their passion is and to meet mentors to help them to make their dreams come true.

You can talk to her about how she plans to do this by sending her an e-mail at Cohnart@yahoo.com Check out her website at Cohnart.com

# What People Say ...

In "The Spring Principle," Susan Cohn masterfully blends her wealth of experience as both an artist and author with ground-breaking research into the phenomena of aging and ageism in America. As someone who has embraced the vivid chapters of her own life, Susan confronts the pervasive issue of ageism head-on, offering a refreshing and enlightening perspective on growing older in today's society.

This book is not merely a recounting of facts; it is a compelling narrative interwoven with personal insights that illuminate the often overlooked opportunities that aging can offer. Susan's investigation reveals a powerful truth: people not only live longer but also thrive when respected and engaged within their communities. "The Spring Principle" challenges us to rethink our approach to aging, advocating for a society where every year gained is viewed as an opportunity for continued growth and engagement.

As we navigate our own journeys towards our golden years, Susan's narrative serves as both a guide and an inspiration, providing practical advice on how to cultivate a life filled with meaning, relevance, and joy. Her call to embrace dynamic aging is timely and poignant, making "The Spring Principle" essential reading for anyone interested in enriching their later years with vitality and purpose. Susan Cohn has not only provided a roadmap to combat ageism but has also invited us all to redefine the value of aging itself.

**Julie Fisher**
**Author**

I really enjoyed Susan Cohn's writing, as she takes us on a transformative journey, challenging the stereotypes and misconceptions surrounding aging with a refreshing perspective. Through insightful narratives and practical wisdom, she dismantles the barriers of ageism, dispelling the myths and generalised assumptions we often make.

Susan skillfully navigates through various facets of aging, from financial planning to maintaining physical and mental well-being, offering a roadmap for living with purpose and vitality. Each chapter is a treasure trove of knowledge, presented in a format that is both accessible and engaging.

*The Spring Principle* serves as a timely reminder of the invaluable contributions older adults offer. It challenges us to reassess our perceptions and to celebrate the richness of experience that comes with age. This book is a must-read for anyone seeking to navigate the journey of aging with grace and dignity, while also being reminder to be respectful of the needs of our older generation.

**Vivienne Mason**
**Author**

# The Art of The Mentor

## The Superpower That Turns Good into Great

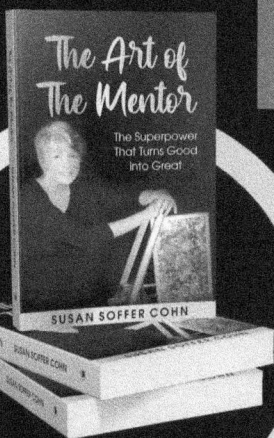

## SUSAN SOFFER COHN

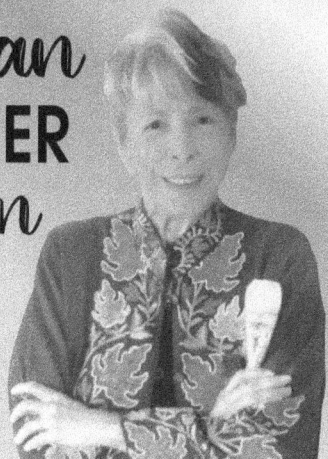

is an internationally known and collected, award-winning, artist. Her work is in collections throughout the USA, Europe and Australia. Author of **"The Art of the Mentor,"** she reveals in her book her journey as an artist who found and finally became a mentor to others. All of this happened after she took her first art lesson after she turned 50. Her work has appeared in Professional Artist Magazine in the USA and Australian Artist magazine in addition to other publications, both print and online. Now, **Susan** is sharing her amazing story and experiences to audiences across the country. Based in sunny California, **Susan's** relaxed, and engaging style leaves her audiences inspired and ready to take on any challenge. A natural storyteller, **Susan** easily connects with her audience and her calm, considered presence is suited to those that are sick of the hype without substance speakers.

**Susan specializes in the following topics which include:**
- How to Leverage Your Visibility by Setting Goals
- How to Find and Be a Good Mentor
- Make a Vision Board to Find Your Focus
- You Can be an Artist Even if You Can't Draw a Straight Line
- The One Hour Abstract (an interactive seminar for any number of people)

*Susan* SOFFER *Cohn*

191

www.ingramcontent.com/pod-product-compliance
Lightning Source LLC
Chambersburg PA
CBHW022052020426
42335CB00012B/664